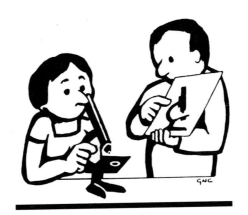

Teaching for better learning

A guide for teachers of primary health care staff

Second edition

F. R. Abbatt

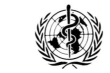

World Health Organization
Geneva
1992

WHO Library Cataloguing in Publication Data

Abbatt, F. R.
  Teaching for better learning: a guide for teachers of
  primary health care staff. — 2nd ed.

  1. Allied health personnel – education   2. Teaching – methods   I. Title

  ISBN 92 4 154442 2   (NLM Classification: W 18)

Typeset in India
Printed in England
91/8923—Macmillan/Clays—7000

Contents

CONTENTS

Foreword

The teachers of community health workers in developing countries have the important task of training staff to deliver primary health care. They work in difficult conditions, often without sources of reference materials and with little or no experience of teaching methods. This manual is intended to help them in their work.

It is the result of a long process of development and testing, beginning in 1979, when WHO established a project to review the educational needs of teachers of middle-level health staff in a number of countries. As a result, a library of some 45 selected books was assembled, and distributed to about 1000 training schools for health workers in the English-speaking developing world, to serve as a source of reference material for teachers. In particular, this library was to include a simply written, comprehensive manual on teaching methods which would help to ensure that teachers could make the best use of this new resource. A draft manual was prepared by Dr Abbatt and was extensively field-tested before the first edition of *Teaching for better learning* was issued in 1980. Funds for the project were generously provided by the Government of the United Kingdom through its Overseas Development Administration.

Since the libraries were distributed, WHO has intensified its assistance to countries through the interregional Health Learning Materials (HLM) Programme. Its aims are to work with individual countries to help them to design, test and produce their own teaching, learning and promotional materials to meet priority needs, and to promote the sharing of resources through intercountry networking. By the end of 1991, more than 30 developing countries had established their own national HLM projects, and four intercountry networks had been set up to ensure the exchange of information, materials, expertise and training facilities between individual countries.

During the past ten years, this manual has been widely used by teachers all over the world. It has been translated into many languages. The first edition had a tear-out questionnaire, inviting comments and suggestions from readers, and all those received have been taken into account in preparing this second edition.

M. A. C. Dowling
Coordinator, Interregional Health Learning Materials Programme
Division of Development of Human Resources for Health
World Health Organization

Acknowledgements

This manual is the result of cooperation between many people. I would like to thank all those who have contributed in any way to its preparation, in particular, the members of the working group which met in Dundee, Scotland in November, 1978 and established the main guidelines for the first edition. I would also like to acknowledge the comments and advice given on the manual by the following people: participants in workshops at the African Medical and Research Foundation in Nairobi, Kenya, and at the College of Allied Health Sciences in Madang, Papua New Guinea; staff at the Centre for Medical Education, University of Dundee; students and staff in the Department of International Community Health, Liverpool School of Tropical Medicine, England; the teachers who read the draft versions; the people who commented on the first edition; and staff in the Division of Development of Human Resources for Health of the World Health Organization, Geneva, Switzerland. Thanks are also due to Dr G. N. Conacher, Centre for Medical Education, University of Dundee, for preparing the original cartoon illustrations. To all these people—far too numerous to mention individually—my sincere thanks.

F. R. Abbatt

CHAPTER 1
Introduction

Before I started to write this manual I talked to teachers about the problems they faced. They told me about the large numbers of students in each class, the problems of crowding in schools, the poor facilities, and the difficulties of providing food, writing materials and textbooks for students. They also discussed the difficulties caused by lack of time to prepare lessons and examinations. All these difficulties are real and serious. This book cannot put right the cause of these problems by giving the teachers more time or money to spend on supplies, but it will try to show how teachers can use the available resources most effectively.

The teachers also told me about other problems they faced:

"The curriculum we are given is very difficult to interpret. We don't know how much detail to teach."

"The examinations encourage the students to learn facts rather than how to apply the facts."

"The students are good at book learning, but they are weak when they face practical situations."

"The courses are at too high a level."

"The teaching doesn't really train the students how to do the job."

The main aims of this manual are to help teachers to solve these problems. In particular, it will explain how to do four things which are very important in teaching. These are:

— Deciding exactly what the students should learn.
— Choosing and using suitable teaching methods.
— Testing whether students can do the work for which they are being trained.
— Preparing teaching materials and manuals.

1.1 Who is this manual written for?

This manual is written for teachers of primary health care staff. It may be helpful to health care staff who have recently been appointed as teachers. It may also help teachers who have more experience of working with students but who want to learn more about their profession.

The manual will also help people who are involved in planning curricula for health workers or in planning systems of health care. It may also be used by teachers or agencies who are preparing manuals for health workers.

A fourth group who might find the book helpful are students in medical schools and training centres who may later be responsible for training members of the health care team.

1.2 Why has this manual been written?

Teaching is a very skilled job. Yet many teachers have little or no training in how to teach. As a result, they tend to copy the teaching methods which they experienced during their own training. In many cases, they have little opportunity to learn newer, more effective teaching methods.

This book has been written to explain some of the basic points about teaching. It is designed to give teachers information about the variety of teaching methods available to them. Teaching is not simply a question of telling students what they need to learn to do a job. It also includes deciding what students should learn, how they should learn it, and finding out how well they have learned it.

This book has been written in non-technical language as far as possible so that it can be readily understood. It aims to solve some of the problems which teachers face when working with trainee health workers. It is also intended to help those people who are involved in planning courses and manuals for health workers.

1.3 How to use this manual

This manual can be used in either of two ways. It can be used for reference and additional reading—for example, during an educational workshop. Participants may also be asked to do some of the exercises in the book and to discuss the work with other people at the workshop.

The other way of using the manual is to read through it. If you do this, please work on the exercises when you come to them. Write down your answers, either in the space provided or on a separate piece of paper. Try to write down your own ideas **before** you look at the comments in the manual. In this way you will get much more benefit from the manual, although it will take more time and will need more effort.

A final point. If you read the manual, try to read through it from start to finish rather than looking at the chapters in any other order. This is because many of the ideas in Parts 2, 3 and 4 depend on the explanations given in Part 1. If you prefer to read the book in a different order, the contents page will guide you. If you find that any of the more technical words are unfamiliar, there is a section at the end which defines some of the educational terms.

1.4 How the manual has been written

The manual has been developed rather than written. Early drafts were reviewed at a workshop attended by consultants and representatives of four WHO regions and WHO headquarters. Further draft versions were prepared and field-tested in Kenya and Papua New Guinea. Copies were circulated to many countries and over 100 teachers gave advice on ways of improving these early versions. As a result of this process of development and testing, the first edition was prepared. It included a questionnaire to readers, asking them for their comments on ways in which the book could be improved.

Many comments were received by the author, and were all taken into account during the preparation of the second edition. The advice of readers was extremely important in the re-writing process. It is clearly recognized that this edition is still far from perfect and so continuing advice from teachers and other readers would be most welcome. The author and WHO welcome any comments. Suggestions for specific ways in which this book could be made more helpful to teachers would be especially appreciated.

1.5   **A summary of the manual**

The manual is arranged in four parts.

Part 1 deals with the general problem of what students should learn. This is an important issue because complaints are often made that students may know the facts but are not good at applying them. The equipment or drugs which they are trained to use may not be available. In the same way, the skills which they learn may not be related to the real problems of the rural areas.

In Chapter 2 it is suggested that students should be trained to do a specific job rather than to learn a number of academic disciplines. To do this, the job must be defined and related to the health needs of the community. This process is explained in Chapter 3. Chapter 4 looks at the job in more detail so that the teachers can decide exactly what needs to be learned. The technique described for looking at the job is called *task analysis*.

Part 2 will help you to choose the most suitable teaching methods. Chapter 6 gives a summary of the general ways in which the teacher can help students to learn. Chapters 7, 8 and 9 concentrate on the specific problems of teaching attitudes, skills, and knowledge.

Part 3 will help you to test your students. This section explains the value of testing in helping students to learn and in helping teachers to improve their work. Various assessment methods are explained in Chapter 12, with examples which can be adapted and used with a wide range of students.

Part 4 describes the ways in which teachers can prepare teaching materials and manuals which will help their students to learn. The manuals may also be used for reference by the health workers after they have completed their courses. It is important that teachers can help their students in this way because there are very few manuals available for health workers, and many of those which are available are not appropriate for local conditions.

PART

1

What should your students learn?

CHAPTER 2
An overview of the problem

- The purpose of a training programme is to teach students to do a job.
- Teachers should concentrate on the essential facts, skills and attitudes. It is neither possible nor desirable to teach everything.
- Teachers should base their teaching on the health problems of the community and on the work their students will be expected to do.
- Teachers should plan courses and lessons using situation analysis and task analysis.

A story

A community nurse completed her training and passed all the exams at the end of the course. She was given two weeks leave before starting work, so she went back to her village to spend some time with her family. It was a long journey because the family lived in a remote village, but everybody was pleased to see her again. Her mother was specially pleased and very proud that her daughter had done so well.

After the first greetings, the mother said *"It is good that you are back because your baby cousin is ill. The baby has diarrhoea and doesn't look well to me. Do you think that you could help?"* The nurse went to see the baby and realized that it was very dehydrated. She thought the baby should go to a health centre, but the journey was too far. So she thought about what she had been taught. She could remember details about the anatomy of the gastrointestinal tract and the balance of electrolytes. She also remembered that a mixture of salt and sugar in water would help to rehydrate the baby, but she couldn't remember what amounts to use.

She was very worried that the amounts would be wrong. She didn't know whether to send for help or to guess the amounts. By this time, the baby was very ill. She made up the solution and gave it to the baby. The solution contained the wrong proportions of salt and sugar. The baby died.

Moral

Some courses for health workers may be ineffective or even harmful because they spend a lot of time teaching facts that are not important. The courses may fail to spend enough time teaching the skills that are really needed.

2.1 Some basic principles

The story shows what can happen when a course for training health care staff is unsuccessful. But what makes a course successful? The following are basic principles.

Basic principles

1. The main aim of a course should be to train students to do a job.
2. The job determines what the students should learn.
3. Only those facts, skills and attitudes that are relevant to the job should be taught and learned. Those that are not essential should not be taught.

These may seem very obvious points, but they do have important consequences, which are briefly explained in the next few paragraphs.

2.2 The main aim of a course should be to train students to do a job

This is the basic principle on which this book is based. It means that if students can do their job competently at the end of a course then it has been successful. If they cannot do the work they have been trained for, then the course has failed.

This means that the teachers must know a lot about the work which the students will be doing. The teachers should watch experienced health staff doing their work. They should ask them about the problems of providing health care. The whole course should be closely linked to the way in which health care is provided. Chapter 3 explains how this may be done.

If this principle is followed, students will be able to do a job at the end of the course, rather than just know about it.

Some people feel that this aim of *"training to do a job"* is too limited. They feel that there should be much more to education than this. While there is some truth in this point of view, the wider goals should be secondary. The first and most important goal is that the students should be able to do their work in an intelligent, understanding and competent way. This is the whole emphasis of this book.

For example, a broadly educated health worker who infects patients because he or she does not follow aseptic techniques is a danger to the community. So it is important that students get the basic competence first. When this has been achieved, other aspects may be added to the training if time permits.

2.3 The job determines what the students should learn

In all courses, choices have to be made about what facts, skills and attitudes students should learn. Choices also have to be made about what details should be left out of the course. It is simply not possible to learn everything that is known about medical sciences and health care. So some selection is essential.

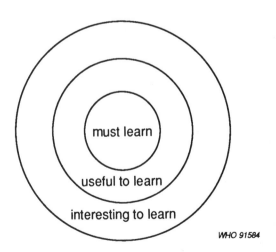

"Must learn" is the target. These are the facts and skills that all students need to learn in order to be competent in their work. Teachers should stress the importance of these facts and skills when

they are helping students to learn. These facts and skills should be tested in examinations.

There are very many other facts and skills that are *"useful to learn"*, but they do not need the same emphasis. Nor should they be tested as thoroughly in examinations.

There are also very many other facts and skills that are *"interesting to learn"*. Of course, teachers should not prevent students learning anything. In fact they should show students how to learn from books, conversations and their own and other people's experience of the world. However, **the teacher's main responsibility is to decide what students must learn and to make sure that they learn it.**

Facts and skills that must be taught are those that are needed to do the job competently and thoughtfully. These are discussed in Chapters 3 and 4.

2.4 Learning objectives

An important idea which should be introduced now is the concept of *"learning objectives"*.

A learning objective is a statement that describes what the student should know, feel or be able to do at the end of the course.

This definition includes some important points. First of all, the learning objectives concern the student and not the teacher. Second, the learning objectives describe the state of the student at the end of the course. The learning objectives therefore do not describe what the teacher will teach or the experiences the student will have during the course. **The learning objectives are therefore a statement of the targets which the course is trying to achieve.**

Some writers also use the phrases *"learning goals"* or *"aims"*. Some writers make distinctions between *"specific"* and *"general"* objectives. The distinctions between these terms are not very clear and are probably not important.

2.5 Making use of learning objectives

The crucial importance of learning objectives is that they define what the students must learn.

They can do this at a very general level, e.g. *"the learning objective of this course is that the students should be able to do the work of a maternal and child health (MCH) assistant".*

Or at a very specific level, e.g. *"the students should know the quantities of each ingredient in home-made oral rehydration solution".*

So the learning objectives can refer to a whole course or to just a few minutes of a lesson—or anything in between.

In all these situations, the learning objectives are **vital** because they control (or should control) the whole process of teaching and learning. The learning objectives determine:

- **what** is included in a lesson or course,
- **how** the teaching is done, and
- **how** the students are tested.

For example, if the learning objective is that *"the students will be able to diagnose anaemia from clinical signs"*, then:

- the students must be taught about the clinical signs of anaemia, how to observe them, and how to distinguish between people who are anaemic and those who are not. For this objective there would be no point in teaching students about the structure of haemoglobin or how to test for anaemia using laboratory methods.
- the students must be able to practise their skills of clinical diagnosis on some patients with anaemia and some who are not anaemic. There will be little need for lecturing.
- each student should examine some patients and decide whether they are anaemic or not. The teacher will then be able to assess whether the students have achieved the learning objective. The students should not be asked to write essays on anaemia, because this is not related to the learning objective.

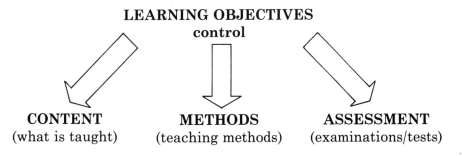

LEARNING OBJECTIVES
control

CONTENT   **METHODS**   **ASSESSMENT**
(what is taught)   (teaching methods)   (examinations/tests)

2.6 How can you decide what are the learning objectives?

The most important thing about learning objectives is that they should be relevant to the job that students are being trained to do. Because learning objectives determine what is included in a course, they can damage all aspects of it if they are not relevant. The way in which teachers and course designers decide what the learning objectives should be goes back to the basic principle stated in Section 2.1.

The main purpose of a course should be to train students to do a job.

Therefore the learning objectives should be based on the job description.

In summary, this is done by making a list of all the tasks that the health worker will be expected to do. This process is called *situation analysis* in this book, and is described in Chapter 3. Then each task is analysed to find out what skills are involved and what knowledge and attitudes are needed in order to do it competently. This process is called *task analysis* and is described in Chapter 4.

These two processes together give a list of all the learning objectives for a course—i.e., the skills, knowledge and attitudes that should be learned. If all the learning objectives are achieved, the health worker will be fully competent to do his or her work and the overall purpose of the course will have been achieved.

CHAPTER 3
Situation analysis

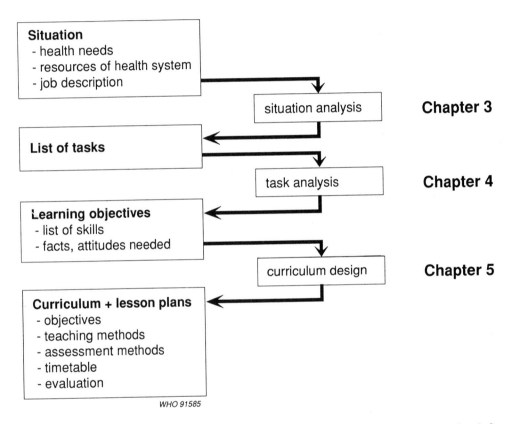

WHO 91585

This chapter explains how teachers can find out more about the job that their students will be doing.

A story

A maternal and child health (MCH) worker completed her training at college and went to work at a family welfare centre as the leader of the MCH team.

One of her responsibilities was to "*work with the community*", but she found this very difficult to do, so she spent her time in the family welfare centre waiting for clients to come. A few clients came, but for a lot of the time she sat and waited. When I talked to her and asked her why, she told me that her boss expected her to be at the centre during all working hours. If she was not there she would get into trouble. Further, she didn't really have any idea about the work she could do in the community. She had listened to lectures on community analysis and development, and the principles of communication. However, she had not been told what work she was expected to do.

Moral

People will only work effectively if they are told precisely what their work involves and are given opportunities to practise during their training.

3.1 **The purpose of this chapter**

The main purpose of the previous chapter was to emphasize that courses should train students to do the job of a health worker. So it is obvious that the people who design or teach the courses should know exactly what the job involves. Unfortunately they often do not have this knowledge. This may seem very surprising. Why not test yourself to see if you are clear about the job that will be done by the students you are involved with?

Exercise

Many health workers in primary health care have responsibility for some of the following:

— managing a health centre,
— intersectoral cooperation,
— community involvement,
— treating common diseases, and
— preventing and controlling disease.

For all of the responsibilities above that are part of your students' work, ask yourself:

What should be the first daily task of health workers who manage a health centre?
What should they do in order to cooperate with other sectors?
What should they do in order to involve the community?

Exactly which diseases are common and which are not?
Which diseases can be controlled or prevented?
What should health workers do to control or prevent disease?

Comment

First of all check that you have answered what the students should **do** (e.g. act as a chairperson at weekly staff meetings) rather than what they should **achieve** (e.g. the health centre team should be well motivated).

Maybe you would like to have a second attempt at the questions.

If you are able to give **clear and precise** answers to all these questions then you are in a strong position to plan effective courses and to teach your students relevant facts and skills. If not, you are like the vast majority of teachers! This chapter will help you to think through the problems so that you will be able to answer the questions better.

More importantly, if you cannot answer the questions, you will not be able to make good decisions about what students should learn. So, the important purpose of this chapter is to help you think through exactly what the job of the health worker involves.

3.2 Starting from a job description

In many countries the ministry of health will probably be responsible for deciding what the job of the health worker should involve. Even in these countries, it may be necessary for teachers or course committees to make clear what the employer intends.

The employer usually provides a description of the work that each category of health worker is expected to do. This is called the *job description* or *job specification*.

So the teacher or course committee must start by looking at the job description. This usually defines various administrative matters such as the grade of the job and conditions of service. But the key information for the teacher is the list of *responsibilities* (which may be given other names such as *duties* or *functions*). Some job descriptions are precise and detailed, and can be very useful in guiding teachers. Others tend to be rather vague and may be very brief.

The aim is to start from the job description and end up with a list of tasks that the health worker must be trained to do. It is usually convenient to have between 50 and 100 tasks on the list. This is not a matter of right or wrong—it is simply a matter of convenience. The exact number of tasks depends on the scope of the work and the level of detail which you choose.

3.3 An example of a list of tasks

The job description gives a general idea of what health workers should do. For example, the job description of an MCH nurse in one country included *"monitor the growth of children"* as one of the responsibilities.

The teachers observed MCH nurses doing this work and drew up the following list of tasks for this responsibility.

List of tasks

- Keep a list of all children in the community who are under 5 years of age.
- Train community health workers to weigh children, record their weights on growth charts and decide when children are at risk.
- Organize MCH clinics in the community for children to be weighed as part of the MCH care programme.
- Maintain a register of children who are "at risk" because they have not been brought to the weighing sessions or because they are showing signs of malnutrition.
- Arrange follow-up visits to all at-risk children.

The list of tasks is simply a more detailed and more precise version of the job specification.

This example shows that *"monitoring the growth of children"* involves training, organizing, managing and record-keeping. The list of tasks therefore gives a much clearer and more precise picture of the real nature of the work—and of what the students need to learn.

3.4 How to prepare the list of tasks

Visiting employers

Unfortunately it is not possible to give a fixed list of steps for teachers to follow.

In preparing the list of tasks, teachers should start with the official job description. From there it is a matter of thinking, asking, discussing and observing until the meaning of each part of the job description is clear and precise. First of all, the employers (often the Ministry of Health) should be asked what they think is involved in each part of the work. Useful questions to ask are:

- *"When health workers start work at 9 o'clock on Monday morning (or whenever work starts) what should they do in order to . . . ?"*
- *"How should that be done?"*
- *"Should they actually do . . . ?"*
- *"What exactly do you mean by . . . ?"*
- *"Which are the common diseases/conditions/problems?"*

The point of this exercise is not to get into the fine details of how to give an injection or conduct a vaginal examination. On the other hand, teachers do need to find out certain facts, such as which examinations should take place during an antenatal visit.

There is a risk that this type of approach may be too aggressive and make the employer act in a defensive manner. It is quite likely that these questions will not have been considered in detail by the Ministry of Health, so staff may not know the answers. The mood of the discussions should, therefore, be of shared problem-solving and not that of an interrogation.

Visiting health workers

After visiting the employers you should visit the health workers in the community and watch them at work. You should ask them questions such as:

- *"How do you involve the community in health education?"*
- *"What do you do when you . . . ?"*
- *"Which diseases can you treat?"*

Again, you are not looking for fine details, but you do need to be clear. It is no good being told, "*I inform the community*". You need to know what this involves.

Asking for advice from "experts"

There may be some experts whom you could ask. They may work in academic institutions such as medical schools or nursing colleges. You should ask them how they think that the job should be done. The aim here is not to get an "official" answer but to find out their ideas for better ways of doing the work.

3.5   Bringing the information together

When you have collected the information from the different groups, you need to compare the answers they have given. There are likely to be quite large differences in opinion.

The next step is to produce your own list of tasks based on these different sources of data. Be realistic. Take account of how much time the health worker has available. (In one study, the health worker would have spent more than 100 hours per week on just one part of the job if he or she had done the work according to the official job description!). Take account of the resources available (such as what equipment is available for health workers to sterilize instruments). When you have completed the list you should then discuss it with the employers, health workers and experts to check that it is realistic, that it does help to solve the most important health problems of the community, and that it is consistent with what could reasonably be expected of the health worker.

This review is likely to lead to quite a lot of changes.

Above all, check that the final list of tasks is precise and clear and that you know exactly what is involved in each task.

3.6   What is the value of the list of tasks?

The list of tasks for a job is the list of learning objectives for the course that trains people to do that job.

This is an absolutely crucial point.

If this principle is accepted and applied many courses for health workers will need to be changed. Students are often taught about facts and skills that are not relevant to their work. For example, in a recent review of one curriculum for health workers, it was shown that more than 30% of the teaching in the curriculum was of no relevance to the actual tasks that the health workers were expected to do. The curriculum was therefore changed to include more relevant teaching concerning tasks that the health workers had not previously learned about.

The list of tasks is used to plan the overall curriculum, including the assessment methods (this is discussed in Chapter 5). However, when teachers plan individual teaching sessions or units of a course they will need more detailed learning objectives. They can obtain these by analysing each of the tasks. This process is called *task analysis* and is described in Chapter 4.

3.7 Summary

Teachers help their students learn how to do a job. Therefore, the teachers must know exactly what this job is.

Situation analysis helps teachers to find out more about the job. Teachers can do a situation analysis by talking to health workers, employers of health workers, and experts.

The list of tasks produced at the end of the situation analysis is a list of the learning objectives for the course.

CHAPTER 4

Task analysis

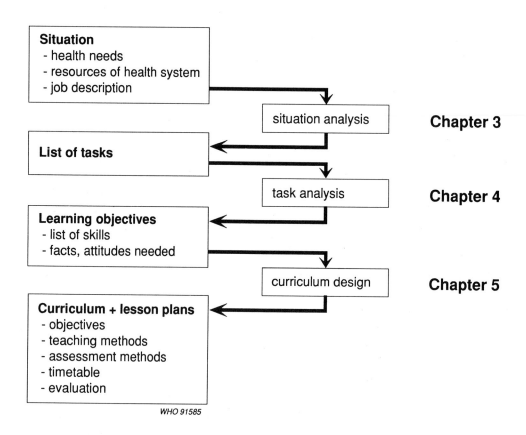

Situation
- health needs
- resources of health system
- job description

situation analysis — **Chapter 3**

List of tasks

task analysis — **Chapter 4**

Learning objectives
- list of skills
- facts, attitudes needed

curriculum design — **Chapter 5**

Curriculum + lesson plans
- objectives
- teaching methods
- assessment methods
- timetable
- evaluation

WHO 91585

This chapter explains how teachers can look at each of the tasks in more detail to find out exactly what needs to be learned.

A story

Mr W, a teacher in a college of health sciences, was asked to teach a group of trainee nursing orderlies about weighing babies in an MCH clinic. He carefully planned a series of lectures about child development and told the students about nutrition and malnutrition. He explained why babies should be weighed regularly and he brought scales into the classroom and demonstrated, using a doll, how to weigh a baby. At the end of the course the students took an examination in which they wrote short notes on questions such as *"What are the major causes of malnutrition?"* and *"List three reasons for weighing babies regularly"*. The students all answered the questions quite well and Mr W was pleased with their performance.

However, when the nursing orderlies started to work in the MCH clinics there was chaos. They did not know how to organize the queue of mothers and children because the teacher had not told them. They had great difficulty picking up and weighing the babies, because they had only seen the teacher weigh a doll. They did not know how to record the weights on a growth chart, because they had never used graphs and did not understand them.

What went wrong? Even though the task was specified (weighing babies), Mr W had not thought in detail about how the students would do the task—he had not done a task analysis.

This chapter describes how to do a task analysis. Task analysis will help teachers to make sure that their students learn exactly how to do each of the tasks in their job.

4.1 What is task analysis?

Task analysis involves looking at some part of a person's job (a task) and writing down exactly what is done. This description is then analysed to find out what students need to learn in order to do the task well.

Task analysis can be done in great detail by professional teams who may take years to do a full task analysis. However, it can also be done in much less detail and much more quickly by teachers. This less detailed approach will still be extremely useful and will be described in this chapter.

4.2 An example of a task analysis

If Mr W had analysed the task of weighing babies in an MCH clinic, he might have produced something like the example overleaf.

This task analysis was done for a specific category of health worker in one country. Health workers may do the task in a different way in other countries. Some may not use the weighing

Task analysis form

Category of Worker   Nursing orderly
Task   Weighing a baby in MCH clinic

Sub-Tasks Actions (A) Decisions (D) Communications (C)	Knowledge	Attitudes
1. Ask the mother to dress the baby in weighing trousers (C)		Friendliness to mothers
2. Check and adjust the zero point on the scale (A and D)	Location of the zero adjuster	Concern for accuracy
3. Place the baby on the scale (A)		Gentleness and caring
4. Read the scale (D)	The need to look at the scale from straight in front	Concern for accuracy
5. Help the mother take off the weighing trousers (A)		
6. Examine the baby for physical signs of abnormalities (mainly D)	Which signs to look for	Thoroughness
7. Record the weight on the growth chart (mainly D)	How to read and plot graphs	Accuracy
8. Decide what comment to make to the mother (D)	Criteria for malnutrition, weaning methods, locally available foods	
9. Make a comment (C)	Ways of communicating effectively	Sympathy for the problems faced by mothers

trousers or may not examine the baby at all when it is weighed. Some may carry out a thorough examination. The example is intended to show how to write down a task analysis. It is not meant to be a perfect model for weighing babies in every country.

What does this example show? First, the task—*weighing a baby*—involves much more than simply putting a baby on a weighing scale and making a note of its weight. A task analysis can show the whole range of skills involved in doing a task.

Second, the task analysis shows which facts and attitudes need to be learned by the students in order to do the task. This also helps teachers to decide which facts must be learned and which are less important.

The rest of this chapter explains how teachers can prepare a completed task analysis like the example shown, and how they can make use of it. No teacher has enough time to do a full task analysis for every task that he or she teaches. However, it will certainly be useful for teachers to do at least two or three task analyses in full. This will help them to think more in task analysis terms and so make their teaching more practical and more purposeful.

4.3 The stages in doing a task analysis

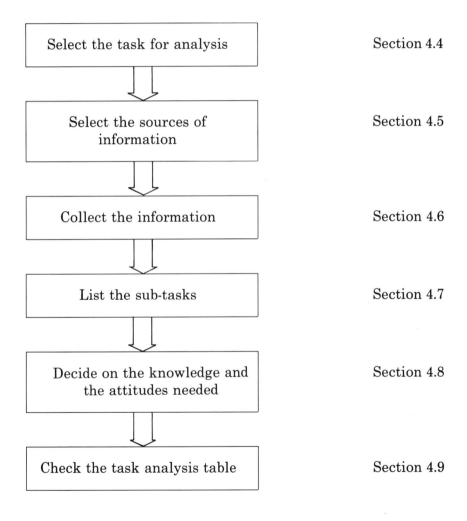

Select the task for analysis	Section 4.4
Select the sources of information	Section 4.5
Collect the information	Section 4.6
List the sub-tasks	Section 4.7
Decide on the knowledge and the attitudes needed	Section 4.8
Check the task analysis table	Section 4.9

The diagram shows the stages which are described in turn in Sections 4.4 to 4.9.

4.4 Selecting the task

The first stage is to select the task for analysis. In this book two examples are used. One is *"weighing a baby"* and the other is *"persuading an unwilling mother to take her child for immunization"*. These are both tasks.

The situation analysis leads to a list of tasks. Ideally, a task analysis should be done for each of these tasks. In practice, this takes too much time, so just a few tasks should be chosen to start with. It does not really matter which tasks are chosen, but it might be sensible to start with tasks that are familiar or are carried out frequently by health workers.

4.5 Selecting the sources of information

When you have decided on the tasks that you wish to analyse, you should decide how you will find out about the way the tasks are done. To do this you should choose one, or preferably several, of the sources listed below:

Sources of information for task analysis

A Yourself
B Manuals and textbooks
C Observation of health workers
D Discussion with teachers, administrators and advisers
E Discussion with health workers

Suppose you wished to analyse the task of giving intramuscular injections. If you had a lot of experience of this task, you might use that experience as the main source of information. You could compare your description of the task with that given in a textbook or manual. You could also check that your analysis was accurate by watching several health workers giving intramuscular injections.

The advantages and disadvantages of each source of information are given below.

A *Yourself*

You are likely to have some experience of the tasks to be analysed.

Therefore you should use it. You are certainly the most convenient source of information.

But remember:
you may not have enough experience or the right experience. Have you been working under the same conditions as your trainees will be working under? Have you been working with the same kind of patients? Is your method of doing the task really the best?

Even if you are able to answer *"yes"* to these questions, you should always check your analysis with at least one of the other sources.

B *Manuals and textbooks*

Many of the tasks carried out by health workers are described in medical textbooks, teaching manuals and guidelines issued by the ministry of health or WHO. A task analysis can therefore be prepared, based on one or preferably several sources of reference.

But remember:
the manuals or textbooks may be intended for trainees at a different level of the health system, in which case the skills will be described in too little or too much detail. Furthermore, they may have been written for different countries or different circumstances.

The tasks will not be described in the form of task analyses and so you will always have to change the format and add your own experience. For example, you may have identified the task of *"monitoring the growth and development of children"*. A textbook will probably give all the background information but it is unlikely to say exactly what health workers in your country should do. It might also describe the normal changes in body weight and the need for a suitable diet. You would have to rewrite these details as a series of tasks such as weighing and recording the weight of children, or examining them for signs of malnutrition.

C *Observation of health workers*

In this method you would choose health workers who are regarded by their colleagues as being good at their job. You then watch the workers doing the task to be analysed, noting down everything that they do or say. At the end of the task you will probably need to ask the workers to explain why certain actions were done and what would have happened if the circumstances had been slightly different. Ideally, you should watch the same person doing similar tasks several times, and also see other people doing the same task. In practice, this may take too much time.

If you have seen two or three people doing the task in the same way, then this is enough.

But remember:

competent workers will be especially careful to do a good job while you are watching. They may take unnecessary precautions. On the other hand, workers may be generally very competent but may not be very good at the particular task you are watching. A further problem is that there may be unusual circumstances when you are watching—for example, the patient may be particularly uncooperative. So what you see may not be typical.

A further difficulty is that you might not be able to identify all the different stages of the task or the events may take place too quickly to record them all. For example, if you watch a midwife delivering a baby, you will probably see her place her hand on the baby's head as the head comes out. In this case, you will have to ask the midwife why she does this, in what direction she is pressing and how hard she presses.

D *Discussion with teachers, administrators and advisers*

It will often be helpful to talk about the task with teachers, doctors, nurses, training advisers or officials from the ministry of health.

When talking to one of these experts, do not ask them what they would teach. Instead, use a *role-playing* method.

For example, you could start by saying—"*Imagine that you are a health worker working in the field. Suppose that I come to you and tell you that I have been coughing a lot. What is the first thing you would do?*"

The expert might tell you *"Well, I would start by taking a history."*

This is much too vague, so you would need to follow this up by asking, *"Yes, but what would you actually say to me?"*

The expert might then reply *"When did your cough start?"* . . . and so on.

In this way you can piece together the specific actions, decisions and communications involved in the task.

But remember:
the experts may not realize what conditions are really like in the field. They may have a good understanding of the overall job of a health worker but may not be good at actually doing it.

E *Discussion with health workers*

In this method you would select a worker or a group of workers who are generally regarded as being good at their job. You would then discuss a specific task with them in the same way as described above, i.e. using role-playing and talking through specific case histories.

This method has the advantage that you **will** be told what is practical and realistic in the field. You will also hear about other people's experiences.

But remember:
the workers may not be using the best techniques because they may have been trained some time ago. They may also have developed poor habits after training.

From the previous sections you will realize that each source has advantages and disadvantages. Ideally, several different sources should be used, as suggested overleaf.

4.6 Collecting the information

The next stage is to collect the information from the sources which you have decided to use.

Use your own experience

Note down how you think the task is done. This will be useful in putting your own experience on paper and will help you to organize your thoughts. It may also make you realize that there are some details which you are uncertain about.

⇓

Consult the manuals

Use them to fill in any gaps in your own experience and compare what you think is correct with the textbooks or manuals.

⇓

Discussion

Discuss any differences between your opinion and what is written in the manuals or textbooks with experts or health workers. This will help you to decide what actions are involved in the task.

⇓

Observation

Check your task analysis by watching the good workers doing the job. Make sure that the sequence of actions you have noted down is the one used by the workers. You should not include actions which they are not trained to do or for which they do not have equipment.

Collecting the information simply means writing down the various stages (the sub-tasks) of the task. While you are writing these down, it is a good idea to ask the following questions.

- How is the sub-task done? Are there any special points to note about the technique?
- What is the reason for doing the sub-task? For example, when

weighing a baby, the nurse orderlies should examine the baby to detect early signs of malnutrition. This will allow preventive treatment to be provided **before** the condition becomes serious.

● What might go wrong? What would happen if the sub-task was poorly done? For example, mothers might be discouraged from bringing children to the clinic if they are treated rudely or have to wait for a long time.

All these points should be noted down. They will be put in order in the following stages.

4.7 Listing the sub-tasks

At this stage you should draw up an organized list of sub-tasks using the notes you have taken. You can write this list on a task analysis form such as the one shown below.

Task analysis form

Category of Worker   Nursing orderly

Task   Weighing a baby in MCH clinic

Sub-Tasks Actions (A) Decisions (D) Communications (C)	**Knowledge**	**Attitudes**
1. Ask the mother to dress the baby in weighing trousers (C)		
2. Check and adjust the zero point on the scale (A/D)		
3. Place the baby on the scale (A)		
4. Read the scale (D)		
5. Help the mother take off the weighing trousers (A)		
6. Examine the baby for physical signs of abnormalities (mainly D)		

The sub-tasks are the things that happen:

- the actions
- the communications
- the decisions.

You should record these on the form in the order in which they occur. So for the task of *"weighing a baby"* you should have a form like the example shown.

The sub-tasks are the skills that students should learn. They are the learning objectives of the course, but they are not the only learning objectives. Other learning objectives are described in the next section.

4.8 Deciding on knowledge and attitudes

The sub-tasks are the key to successful teaching. If students are able to do each of the sub-tasks successfully then the course will have been successful.

So why bother to do a further stage?

The reason is that some of the sub-tasks require knowledge or attitudes that must be taught. For example, health workers must know what a graph is in order to *"record the baby's weight on a growth chart"*. The health workers must also learn about correct attitudes towards mothers before they can *"ask the mother to undress the child"*. Otherwise they may be rude or bossy and do the sub-task in an unsatisfactory way.

The sub-tasks are the *performance objectives* for the course. Knowledge and attitudes are also important to enable the health workers to do the sub-tasks. These are the *enabling objectives* for the course.

How can you decide what the enabling objectives should be?

To make this decision, you need to consider questions such as *"Why might a student do this sub-task poorly?"* or *"What rules or facts must the student know before making that decision?"*

For example, consider the sub-task *"decide what comment to make to the mother"* (after weighing the baby). Here the health worker has to decide whether the baby is growing properly or is at risk of malnutrition. This decision requires knowledge of normal weights for babies of different ages and clinical signs of malnutrition. These topics must be taught and are the enabling objectives for this sub-task.

Consider the sub-task *"make a comment"* (after weighing the baby). Here the health worker may need to give the mother some nutritional advice. This involves knowledge of feeding practices, weaning foods, foods available locally, etc. The health worker will also have to give this advice in the right way and try to support the mother. This requires sympathy for the difficulties that mothers face—an attitude.

In this way, you can list the knowledge and attitudes needed for each of the sub-tasks on the task analysis form. When completed, it should look something like the form on page 22. Note that some tasks do not require specific knowledge or attitudes. Do not feel that you have to put something in every space on the form.

4.9 Checking the task analysis table

The task analysis table is now complete. However, it should not be used until it has been checked.

If you have used yourself, books or discussion as the sources of information, you must check that what you have written describes what health workers actually do. The only way to check this is to observe health workers doing the task in the field.

Remember also that health workers may be using old methods or may not have been trained how to do the task in the best way. So check with experts about the best way of doing the task.

You may find that the best way of doing the task is not realistic because the health worker does not have enough time, resources or training. In these cases teachers have to decide whether to train their students in the best method or to limit the training to what is realistic now. Task analysis does not help in making this decision but it does help in making the differences clearer.

4.10 Using the task analysis table

The value of the task analysis is that it gives teachers a very clear statement of the objectives for the course. These objectives have been worked out from the job description and from watching experienced health workers doing the job. So they must be relevant in helping the trainee health workers to learn.

Task analysis ⟹ Relevant objectives

What is the advantage of having relevant objectives?

The objectives tell teachers exactly what the students must learn. So they help teachers to make sure that all the necessary content is included in the curriculum. They also help them to decide which details can be left out.

Task analysis ⟹ Relevant content

The objectives are also useful in assessing the students. The sub-tasks or tasks should be used as the examination questions whenever this is possible. For example, the best way to test whether students can do the task of *"weighing a baby"* would be to ask them to run a session at a clinic where babies are weighed. While this is the ideal test there may be difficulties in organizing it. So teachers could ask students to do some of the sub-tasks instead. For example, the students could be asked to record a baby's weight on a chart or decide what advice to give a mother whose 12-month-old baby weighed 7 kg.

Task analysis ⟹ Relevant assessment

The final point is that a task analysis is the first stage in choosing teaching methods. If students are learning facts or knowledge, lectures may be a good way of teaching them. However, if they are learning a skill, they must be able to practise the skill—lectures will not be of much use. So when teachers think about whether students must learn skills, attitudes or knowledge they need to think about teaching methods.

Task analysis ⟹ Choice of teaching method

4.11 How can teachers find time for task analysis?

Teachers are very busy and very few will have time to analyse more than one or two tasks. So here are some practical suggestions.

- Do one or two task analyses as described in this chapter. Use several sources of information and check the results in the field. This will take quite a lot of time, but it will be time well spent.
- Think in terms of task analysis. For example, when planning a lesson decide which facts **must be learned** and which are less important. If the fact would appear in the *"knowledge"* column of the task analysis form, it should be taught. If not, it should probably be left out.
- Teach your students to do task analysis. This is one of the best ways of learning how to do a task. When one group of students have analysed a few tasks, they will be able to teach other groups. (This must be supervised of course).

4.12 A less straightforward task

"Weighing a baby" is a fairly straightforward task. It can be analysed by watching health workers, most of whom follow the same sequence of steps or sub-tasks. Other examples of straightforward tasks are *"giving an intramuscular injection"* and *"building a pit latrine"*.

Other tasks are much less precise, however, and different workers will follow different methods. For example, consider the task *"persuade a mother to breast-feed her baby"*. This is much more vague. There are many ways of doing this task. None of them is guaranteed to work every time and each health worker will need to develop his or her own method.

So is it worth analysing this kind of task? The answer is definitely *"yes"*, because students have to learn how to do these less precise tasks. The minimum responsibility for teachers is to teach the students **one** way of doing the task, even if there are several possible ways.

It is also important to do the task analysis because it will often show that the student needs a lot of practice in communication skills and that attitudes are extremely important. While task analysis will not show the **only** way to do the task—nor even possibly the best way— it will show a way that is acceptable and that includes the basic skills, knowledge and attitudes that the students must learn.

Look at the example below which analyses how a health worker might do the following task: *"persuade an unwilling mother, in a remote area, to take her child for immunization"*.

Example

Task: To persuade an unwilling mother, in a remote area, to take her child for immunization

Sub-tasks Actions (A) Decisions (D) Communications (C)	Knowledge	Attitudes
1. Greet the mother (A)		Friendliness, lack of prejudice
2. Find out reasons for refusal (C)	Common reasons for refusal (cultural, procedure, prejudice due to reported experience)	Sympathy, patience
3. Explain why immunization is beneficial to the child	Reasons for immunization, effects, simple facts about illnesses prevented by immunization	
4. Explain importance to community of protection of all at-risk children (C)	How disease may spread, simple facts about immunity, epidemics in community	Confidence in ability to help
5. If successful, arrange clinic appointment for mother (A)	Fully conversant with immunization programme (dates, times, place)	Sympathy, friendliness
6. If unsuccessful, seek an appropriate decision-maker (A)	Decision-maker in local culture (husband, grand-mother, council elder)	Tact
7. Repeat 3 and 4 (C)		

While this task may be performed in different ways, the example given does show some important points which are likely to apply to all countries.

1. The task involves little knowledge of "medical topics" such as types of vaccine or mechanisms of immunization.

2. There is a great emphasis on communication skills—i.e. the ability to talk, explain, persuade, and listen to people.
3. The learning experiences which will help students to learn the relevant skills, knowledge and attitudes are practice in talking and listening, in preparing information material, and in writing reports.

4.13 **Summary**

1. Task analysis is a method for describing exactly how parts of a job (tasks) are done.
2. Teachers should use task analysis in:

  - stating the objectives of a course
  - deciding on the content of courses
  - choosing questions for examinations and tests
  - choosing teaching methods.

3. Teachers should analyse at least one or two tasks in full. They should consider teaching their students how to do task analysis.

CHAPTER 5

Curriculum design

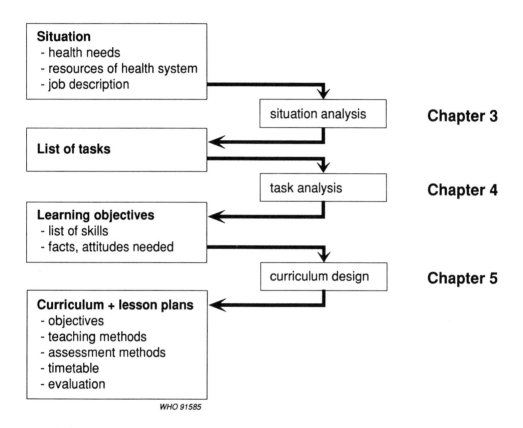

Situation
- health needs
- resources of health system
- job description

situation analysis — **Chapter 3**

List of tasks

task analysis — **Chapter 4**

Learning objectives
- list of skills
- facts, attitudes needed

curriculum design — **Chapter 5**

Curriculum + lesson plans
- objectives
- teaching methods
- assessment methods
- timetable
- evaluation

WHO 91585

This chapter describes how the results of the situation analysis and task analysis can be used in planning and evaluating the curriculum.

5.1   What is a curriculum?

The word curriculum can be used in two different ways. It can be used to mean what actually happens during the course—the lectures, the work with patients and so on. The other meaning is the written description of what happens. This chapter will use *"curriculum"* to mean the written curriculum.

What should a curriculum include?

A written curriculum is needed to help teachers to organize the course. It should contain the necessary information to keep the course well run, such as:

1. The objective of the course — i.e. the tasks and sub-tasks that the students must learn.
2. The general methods that should be used to teach the students the various objectives.
3. The time and place where the students will learn—i.e. a timetable.
4. The methods used to assess the students.

5.2 Lesson plans and the curriculum

The written curriculum is needed to keep the course as a whole well organized. In the same way a lesson plan is necessary to organize a shorter period of teaching. It will need the same kind of information about the objectives, teaching methods, timetable, and possibly some note about the assessment methods.

It is essential to write down the curriculum for a course. On the other hand, many good teachers do not need to write down their lesson plans. There are many good reasons why teachers should record a lesson plan. In practice, time is usually limited and experienced teachers can often manage without a written plan or with just very brief notes.

A lesson plan is a small curriculum.

Suggestions for ways in which teachers can plan teaching sessions (i.e. make lesson plans) are given in Chapter 10.

5.3 When should teachers be involved in planning curricula?

Teachers are often involved in planning the curriculum. They may be involved as a member of a team planning a completely new course or planning improvements in existing courses. Alternatively, they may be asked to comment on a curriculum planned by other people.

They must be involved when they are teaching a curriculum, because they should be trying to find ways to improve it.

5.4 Planning the course outline

Courses for health workers require a great deal of planning. The first stage should be to plan a course outline. This breaks the course down into smaller parts which can be analysed more easily.

It is obviously very important to make sure that this outline will make it as easy as possible for the students to learn. Look at the example below where learning is made difficult.

An example of a poor course outline

Course for community health nurses

Subject	Hours
Anatomy and physiology	90
Microbiology	30
Psychology	60
Sociology	60
Hygiene	60
Nutrition	60
Fundamentals of nursing	210
Community health nursing I	225
Community health nursing II	120
Community health nursing III	345

This course outline has a number of poor features:

- The basic science courses probably give much more detail than is necessary for the job. This means that students waste time learning unnecessary facts.
- The basic facts (e.g. sociology, nutrition) are taught quite separately from their application (community health nursing).
- The separate courses—microbiology, psychology, sociology, etc.—mean that the timetable is probably based on short fixed teaching periods.

A better way of planning the curriculum would be to base it on the tasks of the community health nurse.

Example—A course outline based on tasks

Community health—water supply, food storage and waste disposal
Family health—nutrition and health education
Maternal and child health care
Midwifery
Prevention and control of communicable diseases
First aid and emergency medical care
Training village health workers
Promotion of community development

This outline is designed to train students to do exactly the same job as the previous example, but it has a number of important differences.

- The whole course is designed to give the students the necessary skills to do the job.
- The underlying theory is learned at the same time as the practical applications. This is likely to lead to faster and more thorough learning because the students can understand exactly why the theory is needed.
- The timetable can be much more flexible. This makes it easier to arrange longer periods of work such as project work or supervised practical work in the community. It gets away from the rigid pattern of one-hour lectures.

Base the curriculum on the tasks that the students need to learn.

5.5 What kinds of teaching methods will be used?

Many courses for health workers include too much classroom teaching and concentrate too much on teaching facts.

If you prepare a list of tasks for any category of health worker you will find that most of the tasks involve:

● using the hands (e.g. giving an injection)
● making decisions (e.g. deciding whether a cough is a symptom of pneumonia)
● communication (e.g. explaining to a mother the need for protein in the diet).

You must give students opportunities to practise these skills during the course. Unfortunately this practice often takes a lot of time and effort to organize. It may be quicker and easier to give a lot of lectures, but the students will not learn the necessary skills.

The curriculum should include enough time for students to practise the tasks they need to learn. Sometimes this will involve them in working in the community, for example, in a hospital or nearby health centre. Sometimes they can practise on each other in the classroom. Specific suggestions for teaching methods are given in Part 2. In planning the curriculum, teachers must allow enough time for this practice.

It is impossible to specify how much time is required for every course. However, most courses should allow much more time for practising skills than for theoretical teaching.

More time for practice   Less time for theory

5.6   What kind of assessment methods should be used?

It is important that the course should be based on the job that the students are learning to do. Therefore the assessment must test whether they can do the job. This approach is called *performance testing*. It means that assessment methods such as those based on multiple-choice questionnaires and essays are used less often. Such methods usually only test the students' knowledge. Other assessment methods such as those based on case-studies and case-books are used more frequently. These methods test the important skills and attitudes.

More details on methods of assessment are given in Part 3.

5.7 Evaluating the curriculum

The students should be assessed to see whether they have learned the necessary skills and facts. In the same way, the curriculum should also be examined to find out whether any changes are needed. This process is called curriculum evaluation.

The aim of curriculum evaluation is to find out how successful the curriculum is and to find out ways in which it can be made better. The basis for the evaluation is to see whether the students learn how to do their job satisfactorily.

The curriculum can be evaluated by testing the students at the end of the course. If they complete their examinations satisfactorily, this suggests that the course has been good enough. However, the examinations must be relevant and based on the job that the students are being trained to do. Also, the course may help the students to reach a satisfactory standard, but it may take much more time than necessary.

The curriculum can also be evaluated by finding out how well the students are doing after they have left the school or college and started work.

Example—On-the-job evaluation

In one district a group of health workers were trained to do a number of tasks. One of the tasks was to conduct an immunization programme. After a few months it was found that a lot of the mothers brought their children for the first vaccination. Only a few came back for the necessary second injection.

Comments

Clearly this part of the training programme had not been successful.

There are many reasons why the programme may not have succeeded, for example:

- the health workers may have had too many other responsibilities and so did not have enough time to talk to the mothers about the need for the second injection.
- the programme may not have trained the workers how to communicate.
- the programme may have failed to teach them suitable attitudes.

5.8 Methods of evaluating the curriculum

Analysis of health needs

In the example above, the weakness of the training programme—or the curriculum—was shown by an analysis of the health statistics for the district. This is the best way to evaluate a curriculum, although it may not always be possible. It is the best way because the purpose of the curriculum is to train people to solve health problems. If the health workers can solve the problems, the curriculum is probably satisfactory. If not, it may need to be improved.

Health statistics are usually available for details such as:

— the number of children immunized,
— the number of live births,
— the number of infant deaths, and
— the number of cases of disease.

If the statistics are available, they can help the teacher to decide which parts of the curriculum need improvement.

But remember that some of the things health workers are trained to do cannot be easily shown in statistics. Also, in many areas the information collected may not be very reliable or complete. For example, the number of reported cases of diphtheria may go up because the system of reporting the disease has improved—not because more people are suffering from diphtheria.

Critical incident studies

Critical incident studies are a fairly simple method of finding out from the health workers themselves how successful a curriculum is. The teacher asks an experienced health worker to describe five or six recent events that he or she has not felt able to handle. These situations are the *critical incidents*. This kind of questioning is then repeated among a sample of recently trained health workers. Using this approach, the teacher can build up a picture of the situations that have caused problems for health workers.

Some of the critical incidents may be very unusual or rare. In some cases it may not be necessary to change the curriculum. Again, if only one worker finds that a particular situation causes problems, while all the others report that they can deal with it, then probably no action needs to be taken. However, if several workers report difficulty with similar situations, then clearly the curriculum should be looked at.

Supervisors' reports

In many countries the work done by the health workers is supervised. In some cases this supervision is carried out almost continuously—as in hospital wards. In other cases the supervision is very restricted—for example when health workers work alone in remote villages. Therefore the value of supervisors' reports will vary from one situation to another.

However, all of these reports can be more useful if the supervisors are asked to comment on specific points. For example, you may have tried teaching part of the curriculum differently, so ask the supervisors whether they notice any differences in the way the new health workers do that particular job. Supervisors can also help if they identify the tasks that the students do well or badly at the end of the course.

They may also be able to point out the tasks that are taught wrongly. For example, students may not have been taught about local traditions or how to cooperate with village councils.

If the teacher asks for advice from supervisors and acts on that advice, the curriculum will be made more effective.

5.9 Evaluating lessons

Lessons can and should be evaluated. This is just as important as evaluating the curriculum.

Broadly the same methods should be used. After a lesson (or possibly a group of lessons), the teacher should find out how much the students have learned. This evaluation should be based on performance testing. The teacher should find out whether the students can do the tasks that they have been taught to do.

If the students cannot do the tasks, then the teacher must change the content of the lessons or the teaching methods.

5.10 **Summary**

1. The aim of a curriculum or a lesson should be to give the students the skills and the knowledge needed to do the job.
2. The content should be organized on a *"task"* basis.
3. The curriculum must include a high proportion of time for practising the skills of communication, thinking, and using equipment.
4. Evaluation may lead to changes in the content or the teaching methods.

PART

2

How you can help your students learn

CHAPTER 6

Introduction to teaching methods

Part 1 dealt with **what** your students should learn. This part goes on to explain **how** you can teach them. The two parts should be read and used together, because students will only be well trained if the teacher uses good methods **and** teaches the right skills.

Part 1 pointed out the importance of training students how to **do a job** rather than just **know** about it. Again in this part the main emphasis will be on students *"learning by doing"* rather than simply listening. This principle could be summed up by the old Chinese proverb:

"hear and forget . . . see and remember . . . do and understand".

The aim of this part therefore is to help you to choose the best teaching method for each part of the course and to give some advice on using each method effectively.

The part is arranged as follows. Chapter 6 gives general guidance about problems such as motivating students and making subjects meaningful to them. The three remaining chapters describe particular methods that can be used in teaching attitudes (Chapter 7), skills (Chapter 8) and knowledge (Chapter 9). Chapter 10 brings all the ideas together in a description of how to plan a lesson.

6.1 The role of the teacher

How can the teacher help students to learn? It used to be thought that teachers needed to tell students as much as possible, passing on their knowledge. Now teachers arrange for students to gain experience by working in health centres. They may also advise students to read a few pages from a manual and set questions for students to discuss in groups. In all these ways the teacher is helping students to learn.

Some teachers feel that they must do all the talking themselves. They feel that they are not really teaching unless they are telling the students some new information. But this is quite wrong.

If a teacher gives a lecture and the students do not learn, then the teacher is talking—not teaching.

The following chapters explain different ways in which you can help students to learn. You may already use some of these methods. You may feel that some of the methods will not work for your students. However, all the methods described have been used by teachers. Even if you cannot use a method as described here, you will probably be able to adapt it so that you can use it.

Remember that change is always difficult. It is easier for teachers to carry on using the same teaching methods. When you have prepared a course of lectures, it takes only a little effort to keep on giving the same lectures year after year. If you want to try new ideas you need to work to make those ideas succeed. Some students will find it difficult to use some of the more active forms of learning. You must explain to your students what you are trying to do and make them interested in the new teaching methods. If students have been used to sitting in classes just listening to the teacher it will be uncomfortable for them to learn for themselves. You need to understand this feeling and reassure the students that they can learn from their own experience—with a little guidance from you.

6.2 How well do you teach?

Below there are a list of questions for you to answer about your own teaching. If you can answer "*yes*" to most of the questions, then you are probably teaching well. If you answer "*no*" or are not quite sure what the question means, look at the corresponding section. For example, the first three questions are concerned with "*clarity*", which is discussed in Section 6.3.

Clarity (Section 6.3)

Can the students hear what you say and read what you write?
Do you use simple language?
Do you use visual aids?
Do you summarize the main points?

Making your teaching meaningful to students (Section 6.4)

Do you relate what you are talking about to the students' lives?
Do you give a lot of examples?
Do you relate what you are talking about to the work the students will be doing?

Active learning (Section 6.5)

Do you ask students to answer questions?
Do you ask students to apply information in solving problems?
Do you arrange for students to practise thinking and practical skills?

Giving feedback (Section 6.6)

Do you tell students how well they are doing?
Do you point out any errors or faults?
Do you explain how students could do better work?

Ensuring mastery (Section 6.7)

Do you check that all your students understand each point?
Do you frequently check whether every student has learned the necessary skills and knowledge?

Individualize (Section 6.8)

Do you allow students to work at different speeds?
Do you encourage students to learn in their own way?
Do you use several teaching methods?

Caring (Section 6.9)

Do you show the students that you care whether they do well?
Do you prepare thoroughly for teaching sessions?
Do you listen to students' comments about your teaching?

6.3 **Clarity**

Obviously your teaching must be clear. The students must be able to hear what you say and read what you write. All teachers believe that what they say and write is clear—but are they right? Can your students read what you write? Ask another teacher to sit at the back of your class and tell you whether he or she can see and hear clearly. Look at your board at the end of a lesson and see whether it is set out clearly. Can you read your own writing? If you cannot, the students definitely will not be able to.

The students may be able to hear the words you say but not understand them. If you use words that are unfamiliar to students or speak a different form of the language, it will be difficult for them to learn. Make sure that you talk in a way that the students can understand.

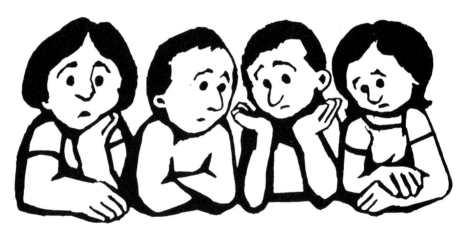

WHO 91592

The students may be able to hear the words you say, but they may not really understand them.

To help you make writing or diagrams clearer you may be able to use visual aids such as charts, posters, flannelboards and possibly slide-projectors or overhead projectors. These will all help to improve clarity. Some useful tips are given in Section 9.7.

Most teachers use a blackboard or chalkboard of some kind. Sometimes the board will look a mess at the end of a lesson, with no pattern to the words and untidy diagrams. Decide **before** the start of the lesson what you are going to show on the board. Then during the lesson, write the key words or phrases in order so that they show the structure of the lesson. Remember that students tend to copy the words and the layout the teacher writes on the board. Make sure that what you write would look good in the students' notes.

At the end of the lesson, summarize the main points—as this book does.

Summary

Make sure that your students can hear what you say and read what you write. Also check that your students understand the words you use.

At the end of the lesson summarize the main points.

6.4 Making your teaching meaningful

Exercise

Look for about 2 or 3 seconds at the two diagrams below.

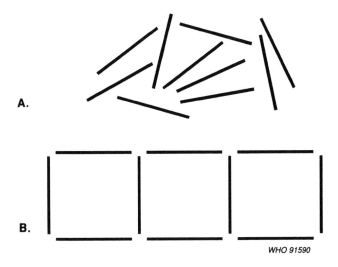

WHO 91590

Now turn over the book and try to draw the two diagrams. Then read on.

Comments

You could probably draw diagram B. It has a pattern to it that makes sense—three squares joined together. Diagram A was probably much more difficult to remember. There was no shape or meaning to it. But in each case the number of lines was exactly the same.

What does this have to do with teaching? The diagram that was easier to remember has "*meaning*". It is similar to patterns you have seen before. If you can make your teaching have meaning then your students will learn more easily.

How can you achieve this in practice? Here are some suggestions.

(a) **Explain in advance what you are going to say.** This can be done by telling your students what the objectives are for a part of the course. In this way the students will know what they need to learn and so they can make more sense of the teaching.

(b) **Try to relate what you teach to students' lives.** Your students will have a lot of experience which is useful and important. For example, when you are talking about sanitation, find out what your students know about the subject. You can then use their knowledge as a basis for teaching. Do not assume that students know nothing about the subject you are teaching. If you are talking about diseases such as schistosomiasis, find out whether the students know people suffering from the disease. If you do this, the teaching will have meaning for the students.

This book tries to make the ideas meaningful to you by explaining them as problems that you may face in your teaching.

(c) **Explain new words.** When you are giving information to students, you will have to use and explain new words and concepts. Some teachers like to use long and complicated words just to show how clever they are. This must obviously be avoided, but you will need to use some new words. When you do, you should define them carefully. You should also use a lot of examples to explain their meaning and, if possible, arrange for the students to practise using the words. This may be in discussion or in writing. In this way the students will begin to get a fuller understanding of the meaning of the words or concepts you use.

Examples of explaining a new idea

For example, you may want to explain the concept of circulation of the blood to students. This will involve the use of a possibly unfamiliar word *"circulation."* It will also introduce the idea of blood travelling round the body, which may also be unfamiliar. To teach this idea you might define the word circulation and then ask students to think of other things which circulate, such as money or traffic.

Then encourage the students to **use** the concept. For example, ask them to tell you what are the effects of the blood circulation. They might say that it allows certain substances to be carried from one part of the body to another. They might describe what would happen if the body was badly cut. In this way your students will quickly gain an understanding of the concept involved.

(d) **Use examples.** When you are describing a new idea or a method of treatment, give examples. You might talk about an experience that you have had recently. Even better you might talk about a patient that the students have just seen, or the water supply for a village that they know.

Note that this book uses a lot of examples to explain the ideas.

(e) **Relate the teaching to the work that the students will be doing.** Information and skills will have much more meaning to students if they know how they will be using the information in their job. You might, for example, want your students to be able to use a microscope. Some students will be interested in microscopes. Others may not be so interested and so will not learn well. However, if you explain that the students will use a microscope in their job as a way of confirming diagnosis of common illnesses, then they are likely to be much more interested and to learn better. The learning will have more meaning for the students.

Summary

You can help your students to learn by making sure that what you teach has meaning for them.

— explain in advance what your students are expected to learn
— relate what you teach to the students' lives
— explain new words and ideas

— use many examples to explain what you mean
— relate the teaching to the work that the students will be doing.

6.5 Active learning

Many experiments have shown that students learn very little when they are listening to a teacher giving a lecture.

They learn a little more if the teacher writes on the board and uses diagrams and pictures. In this way the students can see what they have to learn as well as hear it. But still rather little is learned.

To help students to learn you should give them some exercises to do, such as answering questions, writing notes or explaining an idea (to a friend or to the whole class). The students will also need to practise any skills that you teach them. The importance of these exercises is highlighted in the Chinese proverb at the beginning of the chapter.

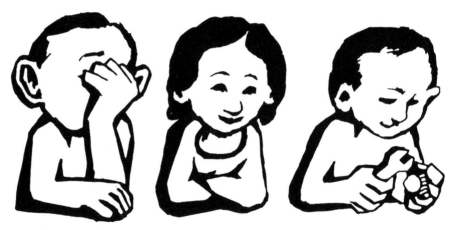

WHO 91593

"hear and forget . . . see and remember . . . do and understand".

Of course some exercises will be more helpful than others. As a rule, the exercise should make the students **use** information rather than just repeat it. Active learning can also be used in books or handouts. To illustrate the method here is an exercise for you to do.

Exercise

Imagine you are teaching students how to take a patient's temperature. Which of the following activities would be most useful after you have explained how to do the task?

A. Read a section from a manual on taking temperatures.
B. Copy your notes from the board.
C. Make notes in their own words on how to take temperatures.
D. Write down the temperature reading shown in five drawings of a thermometer.
E. Use a thermometer to find out the temperature of another student.
F. Calculate the change in volume of 5 cm³ of mercury when its temperature changes from 10 °C to 40 °C.

Write down your answers and give reasons.

Comments

With the exception of F, all of the activities are better than no activities at all. E is probably most useful because the students will need to use all the information you have given. They will have to read the thermometer as well as use antiseptic techniques, shake the mercury down, place the thermometer correctly under the tongue, etc.

Activity D is also useful as some students may have difficulty reading off a scale. It would help the teacher to find out exactly which students needed more help.

Activity C is better than B because the students have to explain the task themselves instead of just copying the teacher's explanation.

Activity A might be worth doing so that any points in the manual which were difficult to understand could be explained.

Activity F is probably not worth while because the students will not have to do this kind of calculation in their job. It will waste time and may confuse the students.

You should not use **all** the activities. Some may not be possible—for example, do you have enough thermometers? Instead, you should choose one or a few of the activities that you feel would help the students to learn best.

There are many different kinds of activities which are useful for different kinds of objectives. For example, you might develop *projects* for the students to do in which they collect data about health needs. You might use *role-playing* exercises in which students act the parts of different people they are likely to meet in their work. You might ask groups of students how they would solve a health problem in their community. All these methods will give you more work to do, but they will also help the students to learn. These methods are explained in more detail in Chapters 8, 9 and 10.

This book gives you exercises to do while you are reading. In this way the book uses active learning methods. Do you find that the exercises help you to learn?

Summary

It is easier for teachers to keep talking during a lesson, but it does not help learning. Instead, teachers should think of activities that will force the students to **use** the information that they have been taught. Teachers should use as many activities as are realistic, and so help students to learn.

Do not just talk—make your students do the work.

6.6 Giving feedback

Feedback is one of the fashionable words in education at the moment. What does it mean? Simply that when the students have done a piece of work, the teacher should tell them whether they have done it well. The teacher should also point out any errors or faults and explain to the students how the work could have been done better. This process of telling students how well they are doing is called feedback.

Feedback can also come from written material. If you ask students a number of questions and then give them the answers on a sheet of paper, this is also feedback. If you give guidance to the students they can sometimes give feedback to each other (see self-assessment in Part 3).

Of course, many teachers have been doing this for a long time, so the idea of feedback is not at all new or different. What are the ways in which feedback can be given?

The first point is that if students only listen to a teacher talking, there is nothing to give feedback on. So feedback and activity go together. To give feedback, you must first arrange for the students to do things that can be assessed. This means that there should be frequent tests of the students' ability to do the practical tasks required, to remember the necessary facts, and to use those facts in solving problems or communicating.

These tests may be formal examinations. If these are held, the teachers will have to do a lot of extra work and the students may become interested only in passing examinations and forget the real reasons for their training. A better way is for the activities and feedback to become part of the normal pattern of teaching. The students will be able to assess their own performance or that of other students if they are given guidance by the teacher. The feedback should usually have three parts.

1. Feedback should give some encouragement and praise for what has been done well.
2. Feedback should give an indication of the overall standard of the work. For example, "*8 out of 10*" or "*Pass*".
3. Feedback should point out any errors or faults and show how the performance can be improved.

Example of giving feedback

You might watch a student practising how to bandage a patient to provide support for an injured arm. When the student has finished, you might say "*Well done. You have done quite a good job. The bandage is tied firmly so it should not come undone by itself. You have also used the right method of bandaging, so overall the standard is satisfactory. But you should have made sure that the lower arm was held level. You have made the bandage lift the patient's hand slightly higher than his elbow. To do this better you should . . .*".

Note that this example shows the teacher giving some praise— "*well done*".

The teacher gives an indication of the standard of the work— "*quite a good job*" . . . "*it will not come undone by itself*" . . . "*right method*" etc.

The teacher also points out the faults and shows the student how to do the job better— "*you should have made sure that the lower arm was held level*".

Summary

Give as much information as possible to students about the standard of their work. Praise the good things, but also show how they can eliminate errors.

6.7 Ensuring mastery

The phrase *"ensuring mastery"* simply means that you make sure that all the students know the facts and skills that they need at each stage.

Ideally this is done at the beginning of each lesson.

When you are teaching some topics, the students may need to have understood ideas taught in an earlier lesson. For example, if you are discussing a growth chart for babies, the students will need to know what a graph is and how to record data on a graph. These ideas may have been taught some time ago, so the students may have

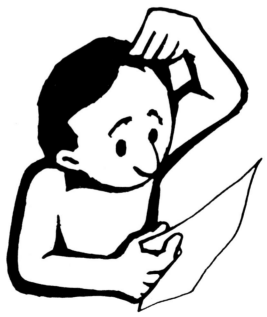

WHO 91594

". . . so the students may have forgotten or possibly never understood".

forgotten or possibly never have understood. This means that they will not be able to understand the growth chart.

To overcome this difficulty you should check at the beginning of the lesson that **all** students know the necessary facts and skills. Do not ask *"Does everybody know about graphs?"* If you do, the students will probably say *"yes"*, whether they understand or not. Nobody likes to admit that they do not know something. Instead you should give a very short test. For example, you could draw a graph on the board and ask the students to write down what a specific point on the graph means.

You should also find out how much your students know at the end of the lesson—or even at various stages during the lesson. Again, do not just ask *"Do you understand?"* Instead ask the students to use the skill or tell you the facts.

This technique may seem obvious. Most teachers think that they do *"ensure mastery"*. In fact if you talk to students and find out exactly what they know, you may be surprised at how little they remember from previous lectures.

Summary

At the beginning of the lesson, check whether all your students know the facts and skills that they will need. Then, at the end of the lesson, make sure that all the students have learned these essential facts and skills.

6.8 Individualize

Most teachers agree that different students learn in different ways. Some students are very intelligent, while others seem to be rather less clever. Some students may be very good at learning facts but rather poor at doing practical work. Others are the opposite. Some students can learn from books, while others prefer to listen to the teacher talking. Other students learn best by practical experience of doing the job.

However, schools often treat all students as if they were identical. All students go to the same teaching sessions. There they listen to the same lecture and then do the same practical work.

Of course, it is much simpler and cheaper to treat all students in exactly the same way. It is also easier to keep control of their whereabouts because the timetable will say where every student should be at any given time. But is this the most effective way of learning? Does it prepare students to take more responsibility for their own learning? Remember that after they leave the training school they will usually need to work and learn on their own.

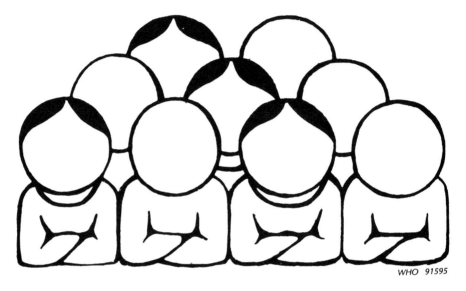

WHO 91595

Schools often treat all students as if they were identical.

What can teachers do to help the individual students to learn? Here are a number of suggestions which would be realistic in many training schools.

(a) **Make sure that there is enough time for students to learn on their own.** To do this you may have to cut down the number of lectures. Some people suggest that there should be as much as 2 hours of time free for individual studying for every hour in a class. This would allow the students to learn at their own pace outside the lecture room.

(b) **Use some different teaching methods.** Some students learn better from books, while some learn better when topics are discussed in a group. Some students learn well from films or film-strips (if these are available).

It is not usually possible to give a *choice* of teaching methods. However, teachers can use a variety of methods and so meet the needs of a larger number of students.

(c) **Make more use of project work.** To do this you set students a large-scale task such as finding out what village people think are their major health problems. Project work allows a lot more scope for students to learn in their own way. It also gives a contrast to the lectures.

(d) **Talk to students individually.** If you talk to the students by themselves you will find that some students are confused by one idea while others find the idea quite easy to understand. You will then be able to explain the idea yourself, or tell the students where to find the relevant information.

(e) **Use self-instruction methods.** Where possible use tape-slide programmes or programmed texts. Where this is not possible because of lack of equipment or suitable programmes, you can help students by giving them written notes. These notes can guide the students in using manuals for health workers. Notes can also be used in practical work to remind students of the skills that they need to learn.

Summary

Remember that your students are individuals. They learn at different rates and in different ways. They have different interests, experiences and abilities. Try to find out what each student is like. Then use this information to vary your teaching so that as far as possible each student can learn in his or her own way.

6.9 Caring

Students will often do things for one teacher that they will not do for another. How then can you use this to help your students learn?

One thing that encourages students to make more effort is the belief that the teacher cares about them. Note that it is not enough for the teacher to care. The students must **know** that the teacher cares.

This does not mean that you should give higher marks than other teachers or allow poor standards of work or behaviour. This gives the opposite impression. Nor should you be content to say "*I care about* ...". Simply saying the words will not persuade many of your students for very long. Instead, the way that you as a teacher behave will show whether you care or not.

Exercise

Look at the list of statements about a teacher. Which statements would you like to be true of you?

A. She wears clean and tidy clothes.
B. He always arrives for teaching sessions on time.
C. She prepares thoroughly for teaching sessions.
D. He shows that he is very knowledgeable about the subject by using all the technical words.
E. She is a very important and very busy person. So she has to hurry away from teaching sessions to do other work.
F. He never smiles or jokes, because learning is a very serious business.
G. She always praises students' work, however bad it is.
H. He talks to students and finds out what their personal interests and ambitions are.
I. She asks students to comment on the teaching sessions so that the sessions can be improved.
J. He ignores the comments students make about the lessons.
K. She requires the students to do work of a high standard.

Comments

The "*correct*" answers are probably obvious. The only statements that need expanding are D, G and H.

Statement D reflects one of the worst things that some teachers do. Teachers should not use technical words just to show how clever they are. They should take pride in the way they make ideas easy to understand.

Statement G is typical of teachers who are trying to encourage their students. But teachers should not praise bad work. Your aim should be to praise whatever is worth praise, but point out the weak points and insist on a high standard.

Statement H may seem unrealistic. Teachers do not have time to talk to all their students for long periods of time. But you should try to talk and **listen** as much as possible. When you are talking, try to find some shared interest. For example, you may know someone from the student's village. You may be interested in the same sport as the student. The important point is for you to show the students that you care.

Summary

If the students believe that the teacher cares about them, they will have an extra reason for learning.

6.10 **Motivation**

Some mention must also be made of motivation. It is often said that motivation is the key to successful teaching. All that a teacher needs to do is motivate students and they will learn.

How can teachers motivate students? The answer is simply to use the ideas described in Sections 6.2 to 6.9. Each of these ideas will help to make the courses more interesting, easier to learn or more relevant to the student's career. Above all they will help students realize that you care about their success. All these ideas will help to motivate students.

6.11 **Conclusion**

Some people argue about whether teaching is an art or a science. In other words, some people believe that the talent for teaching is a natural gift that good teachers are born with. Other people believe that teaching is a science which is controlled by rules.

This part of the book is designed to show you that there are some general rules for teaching. If you follow these, your teaching will improve. If you do the opposite to these rules, then your teaching will almost certainly be poor and the students will not learn.

In order to teach well, you will need to apply the rules for your students, your subject and your school or college. You still have to think of ways to make your teaching sessions have more meaning for your students. You have to be imaginative and think of activities which will be useful to your students. You have to take the trouble to give feedback to your students and to show that you care about their success.

Summary

1. Make the learning active—ask questions, set problems and organize projects.
2. Give feedback—explain how well each student is doing and how his or her work could be improved.
3. Make your teaching clear—check that the students can hear what you say and see what you write. Speak loudly, use simple language, write tidily, and use visual aids.
4. Make your teaching meaningful—explain how it will help students to do their job better.
5. Ensure mastery—check that **all** students know the necessary tasks and can perform the necessary skills before and after each session.
6. Allow for individual differences—let students learn at their own pace, leave enough free time for individual study and use a variety of teaching methods.
7. Show that you care whether students learn—set high standards and get to know each student.

CHAPTER 7

How to teach attitudes

What is an attitude? Think about health workers in rural centres. They may know all about aseptic methods and have the skill to follow them. But when they are working by themselves, they may be tempted to take short cuts and not be very thorough. The way they behave will depend on their attitudes. So an attitude is a tendency to behave in a certain way.

7.1 Are attitudes important?

It has often been said that the attitudes learned during training are the most important part of the training. At the same time other people say that attitudes cannot be taught. What is the truth?

Certainly attitudes are formed or changed during training. This is quite clear to anyone who has worked with students and watched them develop over a period of time. Compare the attitudes of students who have completed a long period of training with the attitudes of a group who are just starting. The differences will usually be obvious. But how has this change taken place? Has the change been caused by the course? Can teachers control changes in attitude?

One of the problems for teachers is that attitudes are not easy to measure. You can set out to teach students how to inject a patient and at the end of the teaching session you can easily find out whether they have learned the skill. On the other hand, you may try to change their attitudes to patients by explaining that they should respect the patients' opinions. But at the end of the explanation it is very difficult to find out whether the students' attitudes have changed.

Another problem is that attitudes are hard to define or explain. Because of this, very few teachers would be able to list all the attitudes that they would like their students to have. So it is not clear what the students need to learn.

Attitudes are very important, however, and teachers must try to make sure that the students learn the right attitudes.

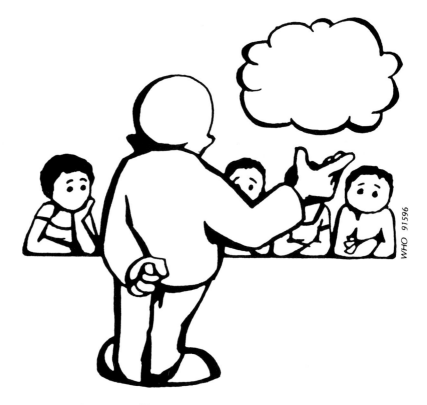

Attitudes are rather vague things.

This is especially important if the students will be working in remote villages or will not be closely supervised after training. In such situations, they may be tempted to take life easily and not work very hard. This would cause a fall in the overall standard of health of the community. This drop in standards can only be avoided if health workers have the right attitudes.

7.2 How to teach attitudes

There are no guaranteed methods of teaching attitudes. Teachers must be aware that all of the experiences that students have **may** change their attitudes. But no single experience can be certain of having a specific effect on all students.

There are five general methods which teachers can use. These are discussed in the following sections.

- providing information (Section 7.3)
- providing examples or models (Section 7.4)
- providing experience (Section 7.5)
- providing discussion (Section 7.6)
- using role-playing exercises (Section 7.7)

Even if you use all these methods, you must be aware that students' attitudes may be shaped by events which you have no control over. For example, students will read books, talk to people outside the school, and spend time with their families. The students will also have formed many of their attitudes before they start their training.

It is important therefore that you try to influence their attitudes as much as possible and that you do so correctly.

7.3 Providing information to shape attitudes

Information is not always enough to change people's attitudes but it may help. For example, the relationship between smoking and the risks of cancer and heart disease is well known by many people. For some people this information has been enough to persuade them to change their attitude to smoking and to give up the habit. For many other people, the information has not been enough.

Teachers can present information about attitudes in many ways. Lectures are one obvious method. Films are often more effective because they can also be used to show examples of the correct attitudes (see Section 7.4).

The important point is to show how the facts are **relevant** to the attitude.

Exercise

List the information you would provide to students if you wanted to teach them about the importance of following aseptic techniques. How would you make these facts relevant to the attitude of thoroughness in cleaning hands and sterilizing equipment?

As another example, what facts would you provide if you wanted to persuade a mother to have a more positive attitude towards breast-feeding?

Comments

You might have made the following points:

- The dramatic fall in mortality rates when aseptic methods were introduced in hospitals.
- The need for health workers to set a good example to the community.
- The ways in which infections can be transmitted.

These facts all show why aseptic techniques are important. They appeal to the reason in students. Sometimes less logical and more emotional facts may be more effective. For example, you might tell the students about an experience that you have had which shows what happens when aseptic techniques are not followed. This single experience will not have much logical importance, but you can make the story so dramatic and vivid that it has more effect.

7.4 **Providing examples or models to shape attitudes**

Most advertising is designed to change attitudes. A common technique is to show an "ideal person" (who is usually young and good-looking) using a certain product. The advertiser aims to provide a model or an example which will be followed by the reader. This technique is generally very effective.

What has this got to do with teaching? Well, for many students their teacher is a very powerful model. Students often copy the way their teacher behaves. If teachers are rude to patients or careless in handling equipment, then their students will tend to follow their example.

On the other hand, if teachers are considerate to the people they work with, then their students are likely to behave in a similar way. Therefore it is essential that you always set a good example for your students.

Other people will also influence the students' attitudes. Other health workers, nurses, and doctors all provide models for the students to copy. You should therefore make sure that, as far as possible, these staff also set a good example.

7.5 **Providing experience to shape attitudes**

Throughout the students' training they will have experiences which will shape their attitudes. They may see patients with sores that have not been treated and that have become septic and possibly disabling. This direct experience of seeing the patients' suffering will have far more impact on shaping students' attitudes than a whole bookful of facts about the need for early treatment of sores and superficial wounds.

The teacher should provide students with as much direct experience as possible. For example, many health workers are responsible for improving nutrition in a community. In some schools the students grow all the vegetables that they eat and look after animals themselves. This experience will help them to have more positive attitudes to doing the work themselves. In these schools teachers also join in with the digging and cultivation so that students learn that manual work is not undignified.

Other useful experiences can also be provided. For example, students should see the benefits of an uncontaminated water supply in a village. They should see how good nutrition can lead to a better life.

Do you think that students should have the experience of cooking their own food during the course—or should the food be prepared for them? What attitudes would you expect the students to have in these two situations?

Exercise

List 3 experiences which you think your students should have that would help them to form good attitudes to patients.

1.
2.
3.

Comments

You may have written down ideas such as:

- Working with an experienced health worker who has a caring attitude to patients.

● Talking to patients about their worries concerning health.
● Meeting people who suffer from some disabling but preventable disease.

Note: It is always a good idea to discuss these experiences with your students so that you can make clear the kinds of attitudes that you want them to learn.

7.6 Providing discussion to shape attitudes

Discussion in small groups is generally thought to be helpful in shaping students' attitudes. Discussion also helps to make the previous three methods more effective. For example, it is helpful for students to describe and discuss the experiences that they have had with patients. During the discussion they will share experiences, so that the experience that one student has had may influence all the other members of the group.

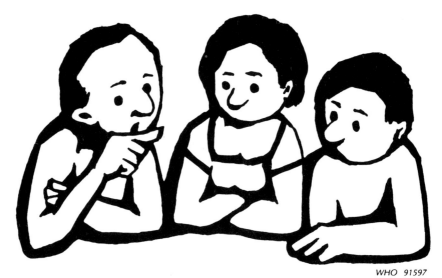

WHO 91597

Providing discussion to shape attitudes.

Another important feature of the discussion is the way in which the students' attitudes change when they talk about their own opinions. The process of putting their ideas into words and seeing the reaction of the other students can be a powerful way of changing attitudes. For this to happen, the group size must be small enough to give **every** student a chance to talk. A group of 7 or 8 students is best and 15 the maximum number for this technique to be effective.

Note that it is **not** what the teacher says that is important, but what each student says. Teachers should speak very little in these small-group sessions. They may encourage the quieter students to give their opinions and have to stop the talkative students from talking too much. But only in exceptional situations (for example, when the group runs out of ideas) should teachers give their own opinions or take an active part in the discussion.

When there are very large numbers of students, it may be impossible to have one teacher for every group of ten or so students. One solution is to let the students meet without a teacher. This is possible because the teacher's role is only to help the students to talk. You can help your students to talk by providing some written guidance for their discussion. For example, you might give them a list of questions to discuss in their groups. You could then ask one student from each group to describe to the other students in the class what happened during the discussion.

Examples of questions for a discussion

Imagine that each of you has been sent to a different village to persuade the local people to build a piped water supply.

1. How would you start to persuade the local people? Would you try to make a speech to a large meeting or would you talk to individuals? If you choose a large meeting, who would you want to attend the meeting and how would you persuade them to come?
2. What rumours and objections about piped water supplies might you hear?
3. How would you respond to these rumours and objections?
4. What advantages would be likely to persuade the people to build a piped water supply?
5. Why do you think some people might object to the idea of piped water?
6. Would you arrange for a piped water supply to be built against the wishes of the village people?

Note that these questions are specific enough to start the students talking and to provide some structure for the discussion. But they also allow students to express different opinions and begin to form or change their attitudes.

Exercise

Write down the questions you would give to a small-group discussion. The questions should help the group to think about parts of their job where attitudes are as important as knowledge or skills. The aim of the discussion should be to encourage the students to talk about your questions and so develop their attitudes. For example, write down some questions that would encourage students to be more careful in their use of medical equipment.

7.7 Role-playing exercises

Attitudes are very important in communications with people. If you respect people, you will listen to them and speak to them in a different way.

Attitudes to people will often be improved if you understand the other person's point of view. One way of teaching attitudes is to give the students some experience of what it is like to be a patient or a mother with a poorly nourished child, or a shopkeeper who thinks that the health inspector is unreasonable. This can be done by using a technique called *role-playing*.

Role-playing is an exercise in which the students act the parts of different people and so begin to experience some of the feelings of these people.

The technique is also very useful in teaching communication skills and is described in more detail in Chapter 8.

7.8 Conclusion

Attitudes are important although they are difficult to define, test or teach. The ideas given in this chapter are only suggestions, because there are no widely accepted methods of teaching attitudes. It is certain that what you do **will** change students' attitudes. It is less certain exactly what that change will be.

Summary

1. An attitude is a tendency to behave in a certain way. For example, a person who has an attitude of thoroughness will generally keep full and correct records of his or her work.
2. Attitudes like this are not developed easily. For example, the teacher must do more than say *"You should be thorough in keeping records"*.
3. Attitudes can be shaped by:

   — providing the relevant background information
   — providing models or examples
   — providing experience
   — encouraging discussion among students
   — using role-playing exercises.

CHAPTER 8

How to teach skills

8.1 What is a skill?

People working in primary health care use many skills. They may use their hands skilfully when they apply a dressing, build a water supply or repair equipment. This kind of skill is often called a *psychomotor* skill.

They may talk skilfully when they persuade people to attend a maternal and child health (MCH) clinic or encourage farmers to grow crops that will improve nutrition. These skills are called *communication* skills.

Then there are skills in making decisions. The most obvious example is when the health worker decides on a diagnosis or treatment. Other examples are keeping records, ordering supplies, and choosing the site for a well or latrines. These skills are called thinking skills or *cognitive* skills.

The names—cognitive, communication and psychomotor—are not very important but are given because you may have read or heard these words elsewhere.

Another way of answering the question *"What is a skill?"* is to go back to Part 1. Each of the tasks defined in situation analysis is a skill. When these tasks are broken down into sub-tasks in task analysis, again each of the sub-tasks is a skill.

In task analysis, the sub-tasks were categorized as *"actions"*, *"decisions"*, and *"communications"*. These terms correspond exactly with the words used above.

"Action" is the same as *"psychomotor"*.
"Decision-making" is the same as *"cognitive"*.
"Communication" is used in both places.

8.2 Are skills important?

The obvious answer to the above question is yes. Very frequently supervisors, doctors and senior health workers complain that when students finish their training, they know a lot of facts but they cannot apply them. In other words, they have the knowledge but they do not have enough of the skills.

What is the remedy?

- First, teachers must accept that their job is to help students to learn the necessary skills.
- Then they must make sure that there is enough time to teach the skills.
- Finally they should use good teaching methods.

This chapter will explain some of the teaching methods that can be used.

8.3 Methods of teaching skills

Teachers often use the following pattern when they teach skills:

1. Describe the skill—explain what the skill is, why it is important, and when it should be used.
2. Demonstrate the skill—let the students see an expert (often the teacher) use the skill.
3. Arrange practice sessions.

This pattern is generally sensible, although the stages cannot be separated completely.

It may be more interesting for students if the teacher starts with a demonstration. Students may need to see the skill being used again after they have had some practice.

Often the skill is described in a lecture (theory), then some time later—possibly weeks later—the students do the practical (practice). This is not desirable although there may be administrative reasons for teaching the skill in this way. Ideally, **theory and practice should be taught together.**

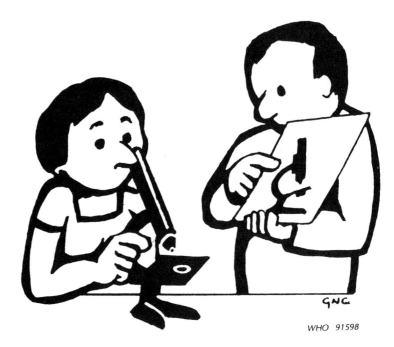

WHO 91598

Ideally, theory and practice should be taught together.

8.4 Describing a skill

The first stage in teaching a skill is to describe the skill. The teacher must explain why the skill is important and why students must learn it. The teacher must also explain when students should use the skill and the stages that are involved in performing the skill.

For example, if you are teaching students how to give an injection, most of them are likely to know something about injections and why they are important. But if you are describing the skills involved in persuading mothers to bring their children to an immunization clinic, some students may not realize why this is important.

When you explain the stages in using a skill, a task analysis will be very helpful. This is because the task analysis describes exactly what is done and the order in which each stage is done. The task analysis helps you to be very clear in your own mind about the stages involved in the task. It can also be used directly by the students. If you use task analysis in this way, it should be rewritten as a list of instructions for the students. Look at the example below which is used for teaching hospital nurses. (Note that the words used are sometimes difficult for students—could you improve them? Note also that this is the way medicines are given in the hospital where the nurses are trained—it is not necessarily the way you would train nurses to do this particular job.)

An example of written instructions for students based on task analysis

Giving medicine by mouth

Equipment

Trolley containing:
— all medicines required
— graduated medicine glass
— teaspoons
— jug of cold water
— small tray or plate for carrying drug to bedside
— receiver for used spoons
— soapy water and clean water.

Giving the medicine

1. Check the patient's name.
2. Read the prescription carefully. Give medicine at the stated time, either before or after meals, as instructed. If before meals, give 20 minutes before. If after, give immediately after.
3. Select the medicine and check the label against the prescription.
4. Ensure that the label is kept clean (if liquid medicine) by holding the bottle with the label against the palm of the hand.
5. Shake the bottle.
6. Hold the medicine glass at eye level while pouring the prescribed volume of liquid medicine.
7. Shake the prescribed number of tablets or pills on to the lid of the container and from there, on to a spoon and then on to the back of the patient's tongue, or mix with water.
8. Place powders on a spoon and then on to the back of the patient's tongue, or mix with water.
9. Make unpleasant medicine as agreeable as possible by giving the patient a sweet or drink of fruit juice afterwards, if this is allowed.
10. Stay with the patient until he or she swallows the medicine. Do not leave it on the patient's locker.
11. Record administration on drug recording sheet.

- These instructions could be used as a handout when the teacher describes the skill.
- Students can keep these instructions and refer to them when practising the skill—or put them into their own manual for reference after the end of the course.
- Written instructions make quite clear what standard of performance is expected. (All teachers and examiners will therefore follow the same standard.)
- Written instructions can be used by students to assess each other and so help their own learning.

These written instructions are sometimes called *procedure cards* or *job-aid cards*. Again the technical names are not important. What matters is that some teachers have found that written instructions are very useful.

8.5 Demonstrating a skill

When teachers have described a skill, they should then demonstrate it. Sometimes the demonstration is given at the same time as the description.

When you give a demonstration, there are a number of points that you need to follow.

1. **The demonstration must be correct.** Obviously you must not demonstrate bad methods. Nor should you demonstrate methods that require too much time or too much skill. You must also make sure that any equipment that you use will be available to the students when they are working in the field. For example, if you are demonstrating how to prepare posters for a talk to mothers in a village, you should make sure that you use only the kind of paper, paint and pens that will be available to your students.
2. **The demonstration must be visible.** All the students must be able to see what you are doing. This seems obvious but often teachers make mistakes here. The problem is most serious when there are large numbers of students or when the skill you are demonstrating cannot be seen from far away.

   If some students cannot see properly you will need to repeat the demonstration. Senior students or teaching assistants may help you here. You could even use a film or a television recording to

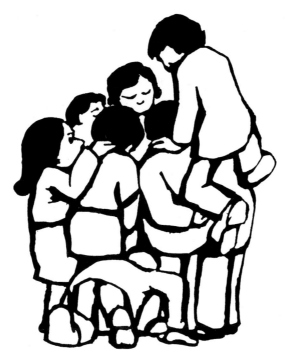

WHO 91599

The demonstration must be visible.

demonstrate the skill. However, most teachers do not have the necessary equipment for this.

3. **Explain what you are doing.** It is not enough to perform the skill correctly and visibly. You must explain what you are doing and emphasize the important points. A handout or written set of instructions will help you to make sure that the students learn the necessary points.

An example of using a handout to help explanation

Preparing for an intramuscular injection

1. Put the two parts of the syringe and the needle in a metal container (a metal pan or tin). Cover them with water and boil them for 20 minutes.
2. Wash your hands with clean water and soap. Rub your hands together in the soapy water until they are really clean. Then rinse them in clean water.

3. Using a swab wetted with a disinfectant such as surgical spirit or alcohol, clean the lid of the bottle containing the substance to be injected (rub hard two or three times).
4. Using a clean swab, rub (two or three times) the place where you are going to put the needle in the buttocks for the intramuscular injection. On the buttocks choose a place for the injection that is fairly high up and towards the side.
5. Put the two parts of the syringe together and fix the needle on firmly. Do not touch the sharp end of the needle.

and so on

You could use this kind of handout in the following way. You would explain why intramuscular injections are given. You would then give the handout to the students. Then you would demonstrate each stage in turn by showing the students exactly what has to be done. During the demonstration, you would keep on referring to the handout. For example, you might say

"Now we come to stage 2. You should wash your hands like this. Note that the water must be clean and that I have to use soap. It is not enough just to get the hands wet. You must rub your hands together hard to remove any dirt and germs. . ."

An advantage of using a written handout while you are demonstrating a skill is that the students will become familiar with the handout. They can then keep the handout to refer to later.

Another advantage is that you are giving the students a record of the stages involved in performing the skill, so they do not have to take notes. This means that they can concentrate on watching the demonstration, rather than trying to do two things at the same time.

8.6 Providing practice in using skills

The most important stage in teaching students how to use a skill is the practice. Unfortunately this is often the most difficult to organize and can take the most time. Despite these problems, teachers must make sure that students have plenty of opportunities for practice.

The main features of a good practical teaching session are:

● All students practise the skill.

● The students receive feedback about how well they are using the skill.

The remainder of this chapter describes some methods that the teacher can use. These are:

— role-playing   (Section 8.7)
— projects   (Section 8.8)
— simulators   (Section 8.9)
— case-studies   (Section 8.10)
— job experience   (Section 8.11)

This list is not intended to be complete, but to give teachers some ideas about some of the methods that are available. Teachers need to find a method that meets the specific needs of their students. They can do this by adapting some of these methods, finding out about other methods or developing new methods.

8.7 Using role-playing to teach skills

Many teachers find that communication skills are the most difficult group of skills to teach, because there are fewer definite rules to follow. For example, it is hard to decide exactly what makes an explanation clear or persuasive.

Because of this, students need to develop their own way of communicating and so, of course, they must have plenty of practice. This practice should be supervised by a teacher, a senior student or a teaching assistant whenever possible.

Role-playing is often used for practising communication skills. In this method the students act different parts as if they were in a play. But instead of words and parts the students are given an outline of a situation, as shown in the example below.

Example

Ask student A to act the role of a health worker trying to persuade a mother to have her baby immunized against polio.

Ask student B to act the role of the mother. Explain that the mother is worried because her mother has told her that the immunization is both dangerous and unnecessary. However, she must be persuaded to have her baby immunized, even though she respects her mother's opinion.

Ask student C to act the role of the grandmother. The grandmother expects her opinion to be followed. None of her babies were immunized and all of them grew up to be both strong and healthy. She believes immunization is unnecessary and dangerous.

Now tell the students who are playing the different parts that the health worker is talking to the mother and grandmother in the health centre. Ask them to talk and react in the way they think that the mother, grandmother and health worker would behave.

Ask the other students in the group to watch and listen to what happens. They should note down things that the health worker does well and any mistakes he or she makes.

They should think how they would have talked or reacted in the same situation. What other information would they have used? Would their manner have been different?

Probably the role-playing will last for only a few minutes. Now comes the very important stage—the discussion.

Ask various students how they would have behaved and invite discussion from the group as a whole about the way the health worker behaved. Ask them also how the grandmother and mother were likely to have felt. Would the grandmother have felt offended? Would the mother have felt bullied? You should encourage the students to think about the emotions of the people in the role-playing exercise. The students should also be made aware that facts are not enough for good communication.

Other role-playing exercises could also be used to help students to understand the problems of communication. The exercise could be fairly simple like the example described above or it could be more complicated. For example, you might add extra information such as the news that a baby in a neighbouring village died soon after immunization against a different disease. Or the baby's father might come into the health centre during the discussion. He might have strong opinions about immunization—either for or against it.

Whatever situation you choose to use, the students will need some reassurance. Some may be very shy or afraid of making mistakes.

It is probably not a good idea to force any student to take on a role until they have seen other students acting. You should try to keep the mood fairly light-hearted—and make sure that the students know that this is purely a learning experience and not an assessment.

While this is a very useful technique in practising skills and giving students insight into communication, there are some limitations. The main one is that this technique should not be used with groups of more than about 25 students. This is because all the students should take part in the discussion at the end. With large groups this is impossible.

A second limitation is that the students playing the parts of the mother or grandmother are only **acting**. Therefore, the students should **also** have experience of communicating with people in the community to find out about their opinions and personalities.

Although these limitations are important, role-playing is still a very useful method in helping with communication skills.

8.8 Projects

Projects are an important part of many long courses. In a project the teacher asks the student—or a group of three or four students—to attempt a specified task. For example, the teacher might ask students to find out about the health problems in a village—or what superstitions schoolchildren have about nutrition or hygiene.

When students do project work they find out facts. But they also increase their skills in talking to people and collecting and reporting information, as well as in other areas. The exact skills will depend on the project chosen.

While projects can be very valuable learning experiences, they can go badly wrong. Teachers must give help and encouragement—without doing all the work. At the end of the project the students should present the reports to the whole class so that every student can benefit from the experiences gained in all the projects—and this takes time.

Projects are useful, provided that the teacher is enthusiastic, gives enough help and there are not too many students. They are very difficult to organize when there are more than about 40 students in the class.

8.9 Simulators

Simulators are extremely difficult to define in any way that is both reasonably simple and complete. It is better to quote some examples. An orange can be used as a simulator for students to practise giving injections, because it simulates the skin and flesh of the patient. Simulators are also used to train pilots how to fly aircraft. These flight simulators are equipped with all the normal aircraft controls and instruments which are linked through a computer to reproduce the behaviour of the aircraft. Simulators can be extremely complicated and costly or very simple and cheap.

Some simulators can be bought. For example, a simulated patient made out of plastic can be used to practise insertion of an endotracheal tube. Other simulations are based on paper and pencil exercises. These may be case-studies (see Section 8.10) or patient-management problems (see Section 12.5).

The main aim of simulators (whether they are simple or complicated) is to give the students some experience and practice in using skills before they work with patients or expensive equipment. They are not intended to complete the students' training.

However, simulators are often not available. Teachers need to use their imagination to think of models such as the orange that can be used to help the students to practise skills.

8.10 Case-studies

Case-studies are paper and pencil exercises which are very valuable in teaching decision-making skills.

The essential feature is that a situation is described in words (or possibly pictures). Then the students are asked what they would do. The situation may relate to the diagnosis or treatment of patients, or to any of a wide range of managerial or organizational problems.

Example—Growth monitoring

Each student is given a copy of five growth charts which have been filled in for different children. The students are then asked to write down the advice that they would give to the mother of each of the children.

Note that this example requires the students to practise the skills of reading points on a graph and of applying the rules for deciding whether children are at risk. The students will also practise the skill of deciding what information to tell mothers.

This example does not give any practice in communication skills.

Teachers could use this case-study after they have taught the relevant information. When the students have answered the questions, the teacher should discuss their answers and give them feedback.

Example—Supervision

A supervisor visited an MCH centre and noticed the following record for injectable contraceptives.

	New cases	Old cases
March	7	12
April	10	9
May	6	7
June	9	12
July	11	10

What should the supervisor say to the MCH nurse?

Note that this example gives practice in the decision-making skills relating to analysing records (a key skill in management and supervision). It does not allow the students to practise the skills of communicating the information in a supportive way.

In this example, the number of old cases should be increasing every month if all the new cases continue to use this form of contraception. These records show a very high level of "drop-out" among patients. This is obviously a highly unsatisfactory situation. The students should be expected to recognize this and to write down a number of points that they would then make to the MCH nurse about how the situation could be improved.

8.11 Job experience

Perhaps the most useful practice students can have is to do the job itself. This practice must, of course, be supervised.

One way is for students to join qualified health care staff for periods of attachment. Ideally one or two students should work with the senior health worker to see how the job is done. Gradually the senior health worker or supervisor will ask the students to do more and more of the work. All the time, the supervisor must make sure that the students are not making any serious mistakes and that they are frequently told what they are doing well, what they are doing badly and how they can improve their performance.

Job experience is widely used—for example, ward rounds and attachments to wards. In some schools for health workers the students spend the whole of the second year of a three-year curriculum in job experience.

Although this method is widely used, it is not always well used. Often ward rounds will have so many students working with one teacher that only one student out of ten or fifteen is actually practising a skill, while the others are just watching. This can be very boring and even at its best is not very effective.

At other times the teacher may spend too much time talking and demonstrating. In such cases the ward round then becomes a theory lesson with the teacher simply giving an informal lecture. This again stops the students from getting the practice that they need.

Despite these drawbacks, job experience can be a very powerful method of helping students to learn skills. Teachers should make every effort to arrange for students to work with qualified staff. Teachers should also explain to the staff that the aim is to provide the students with the opportunity to practise the skills under supervision—not to teach them theory.

8.12 How much time is needed?

It is very difficult to specify how much time students need to learn skills. For most curricula, too much time is devoted to teaching theory and not enough time to learning skills and attitudes. For many tasks, students will often take 2–4 times as long to master the necessary skills and attitudes as they do to learn the essential facts. (There are, of course, exceptions to this general rule.) It is clear, however, that the students need to spend a great deal of time practising the necessary skills.

8.13 **Summary**

How to teach skills

1. It is absolutely essential to teach students the relevant communication, cognitive and psychomotor skills.
2. Skills are taught by:

   — describing the skill
   — demonstrating the skill
   — allowing every student to practise the skill.

3. Role-playing exercises, projects, case-studies, simulators and job experience are some of the ways in which students can practise skills.
4. At least two-thirds of the time in every course for health workers should be spent teaching and practising skills.

CHAPTER 9
How to teach knowledge

9.1 How important is knowledge?

Obviously all health workers must have some knowledge in order to do their job. But it is also true that other knowledge is not necessary. For example, health educators must know which local foods contain protein, but they do not need to know the chemical structure of each protein. Nor do they need to know the biochemical processes involved in the digestion of protein.

So some facts are very important and some are not at all useful. This means that teachers must **choose** which facts to teach. They must not just cover everything in a textbook or manual. Nor must they be tempted to show how much they know by teaching students a lot of irrelevant information.

Teachers therefore need to decide which facts are important, useful, and relevant. Task analysis is very helpful here because it shows what information or knowledge is needed to do each task. (Look again at Part 1.)

In deciding which facts need to be taught, teachers should ask themselves:

"What would the students do poorly if I left out this detail?"

If the answer is *"nothing"*, then the information should usually be left out.

9.2 Teaching different types of facts

So far this chapter has explained that some facts are important while others are not necessary. However, the important facts may be important in different ways—so they should also be taught in different ways.

Example

Take as an example the training of a group of health auxiliaries who will be responsible for running an immunization programme. The course may include the following information.

A.   Whether the vaccine can be stored in sunlight or whether it must be kept in the dark.
B.   How to explain to parents that their children should be immunized.
C.   The date when the vaccine was discovered.
D.   Safe storage times for the vaccine at different temperatures.

Comments

A.   Obviously this is important. Teachers must emphasize this fact and make sure that all the students remember it. It should be included in an examination.
B.   This is also important—but it is more important that students can do the explaining rather than write down how they would do it. This means that they need to learn the relevant skill as well as the facts. The skill should be tested in an examination but the facts alone need not be tested.
C.   It is not necessary for students to know when the vaccine was discovered. However, background information such as the story of the discovery of the smallpox vaccine may well help to make the lesson more interesting. It could be included, provided that your students realize that it is only background information. It does not need to be remembered. Nor should it be part of any examination.
D.   The storage times are important and so the students should be told them. For some vaccines the information may be fairly detailed and difficult to remember. In this case, the facts should be recorded in a manual for the students to keep. The teacher must check that the facts are recorded accurately and that the students can refer to them when necessary.

9.3   **Where should students get the facts from?**

The students can learn facts or information by listening to the teacher. In this case, the teacher is the source of information.

However, there are many other sources of information that can be used. Many manuals are available which contain relevant information for health workers. There are also textbooks, films, film-strips and posters which have been prepared specially for health workers.

Another source of information is the real world. You do not always need to tell students what happens when a sore is left untreated. Nor do you need to describe the food which mothers give to their children. The students will have seen these things for themselves. So they can learn from their own experience. In a similar way, you can send the students out into the villages to collect information. The information gained in these ways means more to the students and is learned better.

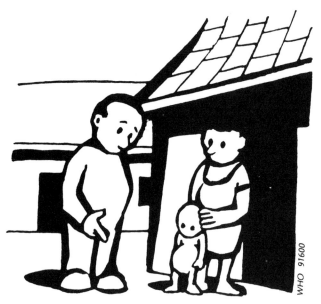

Information from the real world means more to students and is learned better.

Models of the human body are another source of information. These used to be very expensive and easy to break. However, plastic models have now become more widely available. These are strong, usually accurate, and sometimes quite cheap. These models are very useful for explaining the structure of parts of the body. A few working models are also available, which allow the student to practise skills such as inserting an airway. These are useful, although they may be very expensive.

So do not think that you must tell the students everything. Encourage your students to learn from their own experience, from books, from models, and from each other.

9.4 Planning the topics of the lecture

When you have decided that some facts need to be taught, you must plan the teaching session in which to teach them.

A useful way of doing this is to start with the task. Then decide on the main items that must be covered. For example, the task might be to control the mosquito that transmits malaria. Some of the themes you will want to cover are:

— sites where the larvae can be found
— methods of eliminating those sites
— methods of preventing mosquitos using the sites.

When you have decided on these themes, they should be put into a sensible order. (For example, you cannot talk about preventing mosquitos getting to their breeding sites, until you know what the sites are.)

Then think through each theme to decide how much detail is needed:

— what facts need to be learned
— what facts will make the lecture more interesting
— what facts should be recorded for reference.

9.5 Giving the lecture

There are many ways of giving a lecture. The advice given below describes just one pattern. You will need to adapt this and develop your own methods. However, this does give a basic guide which you can follow and improve.

1. **Get the students' attention.** Explain why the lecture is important to the students or tell a story that shows why it is important. Ask the students what they already know about the topic or why they think it is important.
2. **Give a summary.** Explain what themes you are going to cover. This helps the students understand how each part of the lecture is related.
3. **Test how much students already know.** Make sure that all students know the facts that you are going to use. For example, if

you think the students need to know some anatomy to understand a point, check that they do know it.

4. **Present the facts and information.** You can either tell the students the facts or

— use handouts
— ask students to read a part of a book
— ask one of the students to describe the facts
— use audiovisual aids
— show models or equipment
— ask students to examine patients.

5. **Set an exercise for the students to do during the lesson.** The exercise should make the students use the facts they have just learned. This is a very important part of teaching. For example, you could ask individual students or groups of students *"What would you do if ... ?"* or *"How would you ... ?"* Another kind of exercise would be to write notes on a topic or fill in the missing words on a handout.

6. **Summarize the lecture.** Repeat the main points that you want students to remember.

7. **Test the students.** Check whether they have learned the important points.

8. **Set an exercise to do after the lecture.** Ask students to prepare for the next session by reading, doing some specific work in a hospital ward or the community, or revising what they have already learned.

You may think that this is not the kind of lecture that you used to go to when you were a student. This does not matter. A lecture should involve the students in doing things. Just listening is a poor and slow way of learning.

9.6 How to speak in the lecture

You should not spend the whole time talking. However, when you are talking there are some points to remember.

1. **Do you speak loud enough?** Often teachers speak to the students at the front of the class. The students at the back are

unable to hear the teacher and so cannot learn. If you are not sure whether you can be heard, ask a friend to sit at the back of the room and tell you.

2. **Do you speak clearly?** The volume may be loud enough, but you may speak unclearly. You should make sure that the words are clear and that you speak to the audience. Do not look down at notes or talk facing the board.

3. **Do you use simple words?** Make sure that the language you use is simple enough for all the students to understand. This is especially important when the students come from communities where different languages are spoken.

4. **Do you sound as if you are interested?** Some teachers speak in a flat, monotonous voice. They sound bored and their students soon become bored. Vary the tone of your voice and try to show that you are enthusiastic and interested.

9.7 **Visual aids**

Some of the ideas and facts in your lecture will be best explained if you show a diagram or picture. So you will need to use a visual aid, such as:

— a chalkboard
— charts (tables, graphs and diagrams)
— a flannelboard
— an overhead projector
— a slide or film-strip projector
— films (movie)
— photographs.

At least some of these aids are likely to be available. Sometimes the material will be prepared for you to use—for example, film-strips, films and photographs. These can be difficult to obtain, but one agency, Teaching Aids at Low Cost (TALC), specializes in making and selling these aids as cheaply as possible.

Their address is:

TALC
P.O. Box 49
St Albans
Hertfordshire AL1 4AX
England.

You can prepare other aids for yourself. When you do this you should:

1. Keep diagrams as simple as possible—unnecessary detail only confuses the students.
2. Make sure that all lettering can be read by **all** the audience. This point applies especially when you are writing on a chalkboard.
3. Talk about each diagram to make sure that the students understand all the symbols. This is especially important when you use graphs or cross-sectional diagrams.

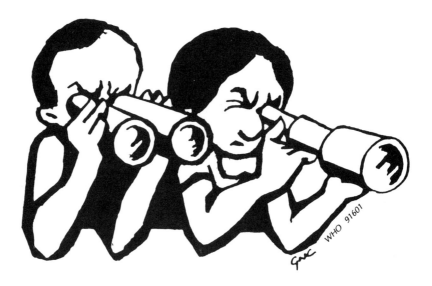

Make sure that all lettering can be read by all the audience.

9.8 Using handouts in lectures

Handouts are one way of adding to lectures. They can be used in two main ways.

- As a guide to taking notes.
- As a permanent record of the facts.

A handout may of course be useful in both ways, but often there will be an emphasis in one area.

Look at the example of a handout below.

Example: A handout for students to take notes on

Malaria

Signs and symptoms:

Treatment of patients:

Nature of disease:

Who is at risk?

How is malaria transmitted?

Prevention of malaria:

The idea of this type of handout is that it provides a structure to the lecture and so helps the students to organize their notes. Students should write their own notes on the handout while they listen to the lecture. This very simple handout helps to make the lesson more active, and therefore helps learning.

Note that the handout also helps to remind the teacher of the main points. Using this framework you could begin the lecture by asking whether any of the students have had malaria. You could then ask them what it was like (the symptoms) and so on. As each stage was completed, the students would then fill in the main points on their handout.

Now look at another type of handout.

| Vaccine | Maximum storage times | | | |
| | Undiluted | | Diluted | |
	Fridge (1–4 °C)	Room (up to 20 °C)	Fridge (1–4 °C)	Room (up to 20 °C)
Tetanus			2–3 years	2–3 days
BCG[a]	1–2 years	1 month	2–3 hours	1–2 hours away from sunlight

[a] For tuberculosis.

This second example is quite different. It provides a record of information that the student may need to refer to later. It is unlikely that the student would be expected to know and remember these details.

The teacher could give this handout to the students during the class. This saves time spent in drawing the table on the board and waiting for students to copy it down. This time can then be better spent by asking students questions to test their understanding of the information. For example, *"If you do not have a refrigerator, how would you organize BCG vaccinations in your village?"*

9.9 Summary

1. Only teach those facts that the students need to know.
2. Plan exercises for the students to use the facts they have learned—do not just talk.
3. Encourage students to find out facts from their own experience, books, models, and each other.
4. Use visual aids and handouts.

CHAPTER 10

Planning a teaching session

This chapter helps the teacher to plan a teaching session. In doing this it brings together ideas from previous chapters and deals with some specific situations. These situations are: teaching people who cannot read (Section 10.7), teaching people who already have some experience (in-service training) (Section 10.8), and teaching small groups of students (Section 10.9).

10.1 Planning a teaching session—overview

The point of planning a teaching session is to ensure that you use the teaching techniques described in this book in the most effective way. You can make plans in many different ways. One method is suggested here, but you will probably need to adapt this method to meet the needs of your students.

The steps are:

1. Decide on the learning objectives (Section 10.2).
2. Decide how to attract the interest of the students (Section 10.3).
3. Decide on the *key points* of the session—and their order (Section 10.4).
4. Decide what activities will be done by the students (Section 10.5).
5. Decide how to judge whether students have learned enough (Section 10.6).

10.2 Learning objectives

In practice, teachers are usually given a theme or topic for a teaching session and allocated a certain amount of time. For example, you might be told, "*Please teach the students about anaemia. There are three one-hour sessions available*". Sometimes more detail is given. This would be helpful but this section assumes that only the minimum details are given.

The first thing you should do is to think about the topic in terms of *task analysis.*

"What tasks will the students need to do?"
"What resources or equipment are likely to be available?"
"What situations will the students be expected to cope with?"
"What knowledge will they need in order to do the various tasks?"
"Are there any attitudes that are especially important?"

Using this method, you should be able to produce a list of learning objectives for the lesson. These may be split into *performance objectives* (the sub-tasks related to anaemia) and *enabling objectives* (the knowledge and attitudes necessary to enable the students to do the sub-tasks). Some examples are given below (this list is, of course, incomplete).

Performance objectives	Enabling objectives
Examine patients for clinical signs of anaemia	Know where to look for clinical signs
	Know how to recognize the clinical signs
Obtain a medical history from patients	Know which questions to ask
	Know which items in a history indicate anaemia

Not—how to take a blood sample or do a haemoglobin test (for this category of health worker)

You should continue this list until you have covered all aspects of the work related to anaemia. The complete list is the list of learning objectives. Note that it is unlikely that this type of health worker will need to know anything about the components of blood. At this stage, you may feel that there is too much or too little detail to be covered in three hours. If so, then you will need to adjust the course. In some cases, you will need to go back to the employers and ask them to reduce the number of tasks or responsibilities related to the job or increase the total time available for training.

10.3 **Attracting the interest of students**

Now you have to think how to make "anaemia" meaningful and interesting to students. In general, students will find a topic interesting if it is related to their own experience of life (not books or previous lessons) or to the work they expect to be doing.

Therefore a bad way for you to start the session would be:
"Last time we completed the teaching on tetanus. Today we will go on to a new topic, anaemia".

Slightly better, but not much, would be:
"Last time we finished one aspect of antenatal care—prevention of tetanus. Today we go on to another important part of antenatal care— caring for pregnant women who have anaemia".

Better again would be:
"We are now going on to another aspect of antenatal care—caring for women with anaemia. Many pregnant women have anaemia and it is one of the serious problems of pregnancy. You can do a lot to reduce this problem and these sessions will tell you how".

A better way would be to follow the previous example and then go on to questions such as:
"Have any of you ever had anaemia?"
"Have any of your family had anaemia during pregnancy?"
"What did it feel like when you had anaemia?"

Other topics will need other introductions, but in every session you must try to find the best way of making the subject seem interesting and important **to the students**.

10.4 **Key points**

Every session needs to be structured in terms of ideas and topics. One way of doing this is to think of the questions or problems that the session will answer or solve. These questions or problems will, of course, be related to the learning objectives. For a session on anaemia, the questions might be:

A. *"How can you tell if a person has anaemia?"*
B. *"What advice should you give to pregnant women to prevent them becoming anaemic?"*
C. *"What is anaemia?"*

D. *"How can it be treated?"*

E. *"Why is anaemia important?"*

When you have listed all the key points or questions, you should then try to put them into a sensible order.

Exercise

What order would you choose? For example, if you would teach point E first, put the letter E beside number 1, below.

1.

2.

3.

4.

5.

Comments

Probably you have put them in the order C, E, A, D, B. However, the various points could also be taught in a different order.

The overall pattern of the session is now established. There will be an introduction designed to gain the students' interest. This will be followed by the main part of the session dealing with the key points in order. Finally there will be a summary.

10.5 **Activities**

Often teachers think mainly about what they will do during a session. This is natural, but it is better for teachers to think about what the students will do. As discussed in Section 6.5, students learn very much faster when they are active.

How could "anaemia" be made active?

The starting point is to go back to the objectives. Certainly students will have to practise all of the performance objectives. In this case the students should, as a minimum, look at each other's conjunctivas and practise checking for the other clinical signs. Ideally, they should then go on to examine patients. However, they could be asked to do exercises based on case-studies which describe different patients, some of whom have anaemia and some who do not. Role-playing exercises could also be used for the students to practise giving advice to mothers about anaemia.

It is also important to try to make the learning of facts as active as possible. This can be done very simply by setting a short test at the end of the session. Another and possibly better way is to ask the students questions during the session. Do not tell the students everything. Encourage them to think, deduce or guess what the facts are. The less the teacher **tells** and the more the students **work out for themselves** the better.

Incidentally, when you ask a question, it is much better to ask **all** students to write down their answer on a piece of paper than to ask only one student to speak the answer. This gives you a chance to look at all the answers and so judge how well the students are doing. It also makes **every** student active instead of just one.

10.6 **Judging how much students have learned**

An integral part of all teaching sessions should be some form of assessment. Teachers should not assume that everything they say has been learned. The activities described above also allow teachers to judge whether the students have achieved a good enough standard.

Ideally, you should only begin teaching a new group of topics when all the students have achieved all the learning objectives related to the previous session. This is rarely achieved in practice. However, the principle is clear and you should try to follow it as closely as possible. You will only know whether you are doing this if you assess what the students have learned.

10.7 **Teaching people who cannot read**

Many health workers cannot read or find reading and writing very difficult because they have had little or no schooling. The following points may help you to train people with such difficulties.

- Many people who cannot read are just as intelligent and capable of learning as other people. They simply did not have the chance to learn how to read and write when they were children. So they must not be treated as stupid or slow.

- There will be no point in providing these students with written textbooks or written handouts—or writing words on the board.
- The students may find pictures just as difficult to understand as words. However, pictures can be meaningful if they are explained. They can help students to remember what you have said.
- It is especially important to make learning as active as possible. You should draw on the experience and communication skills of the students. Keep asking them what they already know and what they would do in certain situations.

10.8 In-service training

The purpose of in-service training should be to improve the way in which health workers do their work. This is a fundamental point which is often ignored. As a result refresher training is given, which has no impact at all on the way in which the work is done.

How can you avoid this problem?

First, you need to think carefully about exactly what improvement in working methods is required. You will need to talk to managers and supervisors. You will also need to go to the field and observe the way in which health workers do their work. In this way you can prepare a list of tasks that should be done differently.

Then you should give some thought to the reasons why the tasks are being done badly.

- Is it because the health workers do not know what should be done?
- Is it because they do not have the necessary skills?
- Is it because they are being forced to work in the wrong way?
- Is it because they do not have the right equipment or supplies—or enough time to do the task correctly?

If the reasons are related to a shortage of supplies or other factors outside the control of the health workers, then in-service training for health workers will not improve the situation.

Take a different situation. The health workers are giving antibiotics to children with a common cold. You find that they are doing this because the parents insist that their children should be given antibiotics and will make complaints if the children do not get them. To solve this problem, you might need to train the health workers in ways of explaining to the parents why antibiotics would be of no use. Certainly, just telling health workers when to give antibiotics would not have much impact.

This process of analysis will lead to a set of learning objectives. They should be very specific and designed to lead to changes in working methods that are realistic and that will improve the quality of health care. General refresher courses covering a lot of topics, but not dealing with anything in much depth, should not take place.

A final point about in-service training courses concerns the teaching methods. Most of the health workers will be experienced and already have a lot of knowledge and skill. This must be recognized. You should make a point of **asking** them what they would do to improve situations, rather than **telling** them. Health workers usually know much more than teachers about how health care can be provided in the field situation.

10.9 **Working with groups of students**

Much has been said and written about the advantages of small-group teaching. There are indeed many potential advantages. Unfortunately these advantages are not always apparent because teachers may not use the methods effectively.

One problem is that small groups are sometimes taught in exactly the same way as large groups. The same sort of lecturing style is used. The only difference is that fewer people hear the lecture. If this happens, very little benefit can be expected.

At the other extreme, some teachers have such confidence in the use of group discussions that they give the group a topic to discuss and leave them to discuss it in their own way. Usually this leads to a very disorganized discussion:

— nobody knows who is right and who is wrong,
— the confident, assertive students talk all the time while the shy students never speak,
— the students do not listen to what other students say,
— topics are changed more or less at random.

Where this happens, very little learning occurs.

In order to avoid these two extremes, you should:

- Have a very clear idea before the session begins concerning the topics to be discussed and the activities that the group will take part in.
- Control the discussion by encouraging the shy people to give their ideas first and by ensuring that all students have some chance to give their views.
- Control the discussion by ensuring that all students keep to the topic being discussed, by pointing out differences (or similarities) between the ideas given by different people, and by ensuring that the discussion is summarized in writing.
- Give feedback to ensure that all students know whether the opinions or ideas given are right or wrong.
- Tell students when they make points that are wrong. This must be done in such a way that they are not discouraged.
- Encourage a group spirit by setting tasks for the students to work on as a group.

If these rules are followed, small groups can learn quickly because all the students are actively involved in thinking and in expressing their ideas.

PART
3

Finding out how much your students have learned

CHAPTER 11

General issues in assessment

One of the most important parts of the teacher's job is to find out how much students have learned. This process is called assessment. It can be carried out by setting examinations or watching students at work. This chapter covers the general issues and problems related to specific methods of assessment.

11.1 Why must students be assessed?

Most teachers agree that students should take some kind of examination or that students' ability should be measured in some way. In other words, students should be assessed.

It is important to assess students because:

1. Teachers need to make sure that the students will be able to do the job competently. This is especially important in all the health professions.
2. Examinations and tests encourage students to work harder.
3. Assessments can be used to guide teachers and students about which parts of the course have been successful and which parts need to be improved.

Naturally no single assessment during the course can achieve all these objectives. For example, a final examination may be good for seeing whether students are able to do the job. But it will not be much use in guiding students about what they should learn.

It is important to think about the reason **why** you are assessing students in any test or examination. Then you can design the test accordingly. You need to decide who will do the assessing, when it will be done, and what kinds of questions you will use.

11.2 **What makes a good assessment?**

When you design the assessment methods for a course or lesson, there are five questions that you need to consider.

1. Does the assessment comply with the regulations for the course?
2. Is the assessment reasonably economical in terms of materials and time?
3. Does the assessment test the important skills and abilities? (*Is the method valid?*)
4. Are you sure that the marks gained by each student are accurate? (*Is the marking reliable?*)
5. Does the assessment give information that will help the students to learn better and help you to improve your teaching?

The first two points are fairly straightforward. Sometimes there are regulations about the kinds of examinations that must be used. These regulations must be observed, but often the regulations only concern the final examinations and allow teachers to choose which methods of assessment to use during the course. If you feel that the regulations prevent you assessing the students in a satisfactory way, talk to other teachers and the people responsible for making the regulations. They may decide that the regulations need to be changed.

Assessments must not involve too much time and effort. Methods such as oral examinations and essays have disadvantages because they take up so much of the teachers' and examiners' time.

The remaining questions are discussed in Sections 11.3–11.5.

11.3 **Making sure that the assessment tests the important skills and abilities**

After some recent anatomy and physiology examinations in a medical school, a senior clinician said "*I could not answer the questions, nor could any of the other doctors who read the examination paper. I could not understand why the students needed to know these things.*"

This case highlights a serious problem that can occur in any schools that train health workers—students are often asked about facts that are not important.

This problem is serious because students naturally want to do well in examinations and so they learn what they think will be in the examination. The solution is to test **only** those skills and abilities that you believe are important.

If the learning objectives have been derived properly, then all the learning objectives will be important. Therefore **the assessment should test directly whether the learning objectives have been achieved**. If this is done, then the assessment will test the important skills and abilities. When this happens, the assessment is said to be *valid*.

Sometimes examinations focus mainly on knowledge and tend to ignore the performance of students. This is bad. For example, consider one of the tasks of health educators—*"persuade mothers to breast-feed their babies"*. In a bad examination, health educators might be asked to write essays on the nutritional value of breast milk. This assessment would only test a few of the skills needed (it does not cover the skills of talking to mothers) and so it is not valid.

It is easy to advise teachers to make examinations valid by testing the performance of their students. It is much more difficult for the teachers to plan assessments that will do this. Some ideas are given in Chapter 12.

11.4 Making assessment reliable

In a recent examination, the students were asked to write an essay about the treatment of burns. The papers were marked by the teacher who had taught the course. Then another teacher marked the same examination papers. The scores given by the two teachers were very different. For example, one student was given 45% by one teacher (a fail) and 70% by the other.

This demonstrates that in this examination the marking was not *reliable*.

Clearly, the final mark should be reliable or it becomes meaningless. How can you be sure that a mark is reliable? The answer is to try to cut out the errors involved in the assessment process. Use assessment methods that are less likely to lead to errors. (For example, the marking of multiple-choice questions is more reliable than that of essays.)

You should also use techniques that help the people marking the examination to work to a uniform standard. These methods are described in more detail in Chapter 12.

11.5 Using assessment to help students to learn

Tests and examinations can encourage students to do more work — and so they help them to learn. However, assessment can also show students exactly what they need to spend more time on. In many courses the teachers give frequent tests and then tell the students what exactly they have done badly. In this way students get feedback about the quality of their work and can improve their performance.

To illustrate this point, look at the results for five students who took a 4-part test in the middle of a course.

Exercise: Using assessment to help students to learn

Student	Part 1	Part 2	Part 3	Part 4
A	√	×	×	√
B	√	√	×	√
C	√	√	√	√
D	√	√	×	×
E	√	√	×	×

√— satisfactory standard
×— unsatisfactory standard.

What would you do if you were the teacher?

Comments

Probably you would be satisfied with Part 1. For Part 2, you should advise student A that his standard was not good enough. You should explain why the work was not good and how it could be made better. Ideally the student should be tested again on this part at a later date.

The results for Part 3 show that only one student reached a satisfactory standard. Probably this part needs to be taught again. Here the teacher gets feedback about his or her own performance—so perhaps next year the topic will be taught differently.

Part 4 shows that two students need more guidance. However, it would probably be a waste of time to repeat Part 4 for the whole class.

If you do everything suggested in the comments above, you will find that it will take you a lot of time to assess students. This is a problem, but giving students this kind of individual guidance is one of the most valuable things that a teacher can do. You must try to make time. One way is to spend less time lecturing to the class and instead to let students learn directly from manuals, handouts and practical experience.

Note that this frequent testing and guidance applies equally well to both the knowledge and the skills that need to be learned.

11.6 **Continuous assessment**

In some courses, students sit one final examination at the end of the course. In other courses, students work under constant supervision. Between these two extremes, there are courses with tests or assessments every week, month or term. This type of assessment is usually called "continuous assessment", although "frequent assessment" would be a more accurate description.

What are the advantages of continuous assessment?

- Because there are several assessments, an error in any one assessment is less important. Continuous assessment tends to be more reliable.
- The tensions and worries of the single final examination are reduced.
- Because students are assessed throughout the course, they tend to work harder during the course instead of making a single desperate effort at the end.
- If students do poorly in one test, they have time to correct their errors before the end of the course. Continuous assessment gives more guidance to both teachers and students.
- Students are shown throughout the course what standard is expected.

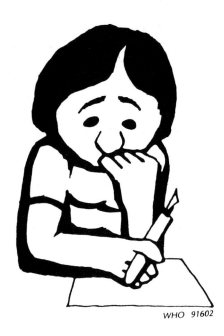

WHO 91602

The tensions and worries of a single final examination.

Of course there are some disadvantages as well. The main disadvantage is that continuous assessment takes more time and effort for teachers to organize.

Continuous assessment can take many forms. It may be a series of written tests. It may involve observation of students while they are working on a ward, in the laboratory or in the field. The marks given may be recorded to decide whether students eventually pass or fail. Or the marks may be used only to guide students. Whatever system is followed, continuous assessment offers important advantages both in helping students to learn and in making more accurate and reliable judgements about how much they have learned.

11.7 **Self-assessment**

Self-assessment is the name given to assessment where students assess their own performance.

Some teachers are very worried by this idea because they feel that students are not responsible enough or do not know enough. This is probably true at the beginning of the course. However, some health workers will be working with very little supervision after they have qualified. So in the job they **must** assess themselves. Therefore it is a good idea to give the students some experience of self-assessment while they are still being trained.

Naturally self-assessment is a method that is used for only part of the time. Teachers or external examiners will be used to decide whether students should pass or fail at the end of a course. However, self-assessment can be used during the course. It will help to save time and give students a greater sense of responsibility.

In self-assessment, students need clear guidance about what standards are required. They must also be given a very clear idea of the task. For example, you might ask students to:

1. Inspect 50 microscope slides of blood samples to determine whether malaria parasites are present.
2. Fill in standard forms for stock control in a pharmacy.
3. Plot a patient's temperature on a chart.
4. Weigh and record the approximate weight of a baby.

In all these examples, the students can compare their own work with a correct answer and so learn whether their work is satisfactory. Note that cheating is not a problem, because the purpose of self-assessment is to learn—not to score points in an examination.

11.8 **Peer-assessment**

An alternative to self-assessment is peer-assessment. This is the name given to assessment where students assess each other.

This method is not suitable for deciding whether students pass or fail at the end of a course. But it is a very good method for helping students to learn.

Many students ask a friend to test them when they are revising for an examination. This practice can be encouraged and guided by the teacher. For example, you could give the students written instructions for doing a job. Then one of the students attempts to do the job, while the other one watches and comments. The students then change over and the second student does the job watched by the first one.

You must of course provide the written instructions. These can be prepared either from your own experience or from a manual.

Peer-assessment can help to make field experience have more meaning and relevance for students. Instead of vaguely trying to

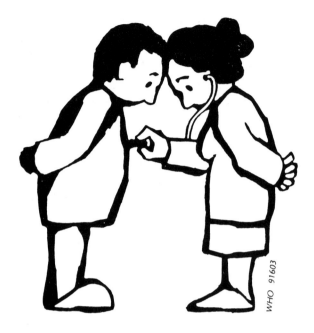

WHO 91603

"Then one of the students attempts to do the job . . .".

do a job as well as possible, each student will be supervised by a
fellow student who is there to watch and advise.

11.9 **Summary**

Exercise

Look at the three examples of assessment methods given below. Then comment on them using some of the points made in Section 11.2:

— Is the assessment economical in terms of materials and time?
— Does the assessment test the important skills and abilities? (Is it valid?)
— Are the marks accurate (reliable)?
— Does the assessment help students to learn?

Now look at the following examples.

A. At the end of the course, a written examination is held in which the students have to write four essays in 3 hours. Then an external examiner meets all the students individually for 15 minutes to give them an oral examination on what they have learned.
B. Every 2 weeks during the course, students have to answer 20 multiple-choice questions on topics such as signs and symptoms of diseases, methods of treatment, and prevention of disease. The students mark the papers themselves by comparing the answers with the correct answers supplied by the teacher.
C. Trainee community health nurses (CHNs) spend 1 month working with an experienced CHN (two students work with each CHN). The students do most of the work themselves under supervision. The supervisor then writes a report on the students.

Write down your comments on each assessment method.

Comments

Method	Economy of time	Validity	Reliability	Helping learning
A	Poor	Poor	Poor	Poor
B	Good—after 1st year	Misses many important skills	Very good	Good
C	Poor	Very good	Moderate	Good

A. This method is bad in almost every way. It will take a long time to mark the essays and to conduct the oral examinations. Students will not have to write essays or talk to external examiners after the course—so the skills tested are not important. Essay-marking and marks given in oral examinations are frequently **not** reliable. The timing of the examination also means that students will not learn much from it.
B. It will take a lot of time to set the multiple-choice questions. But the questions can be used year after year (with a few changes) and they are very quick to mark. The assessment may test important skills, depending on the exact questions asked and what work the students are being trained to do. However, multiple-choice questions usually only test factual knowledge, so they cannot test many of the important skills that should be tested. The

reliability is excellent—there should be very few marking errors. Students should learn both from marking each other's work and from seeing exactly what errors they have made. But note that it will only help them to learn factual knowledge.

C. This method will take quite a lot of time because the supervisor writes individual reports. However, the important skills are being tested. The reliability may be low because different supervisors may have different standards. The assessment should help learning very effectively.

These examples illustrate that each assessment method has some disadvantages. You should be aware of these problems and try to reduce them as far as possible. Specific guidance on different assessment methods is given in Chapter 12.

Assessment methods

The previous chapter discussed the general issues related to the assessment of students. This chapter describes specific methods that will help to improve the way you assess your students. Examples of each method are given and their advantages and disadvantages are discussed.

12.1 Oral examinations

In an oral examination, each student is interviewed by one or two examiners. Usually students are asked to tell the examiner what they know about some topic or what they would do in some situation that might happen in their job.

The main advantages of oral examinations are that the examiner can ask for more detailed information and can probe to find out how much each student knows.

However, this is not a very satisfactory method of assessment. Students are often made extremely anxious by examiners, even though the examiners try to be friendly. This is unfair on the students, because they will not face this kind of stress in their job. Many students get worse results in oral examinations than they deserve. Oral examinations also take up a lot of time and are often criticized because the marking is unreliable. Further, oral examinations rarely test the important skills and do not usually help students to learn.

You should **not** use oral examinations to assess students unless you have some specific reason for doing so.

12.2 Essays

Essays have been widely used in assessing students in the health professions. But again, this method has very serious disadvantages.

In one course, students were asked to write an essay on polio immunization. This is a very poor test even though the topic was of some relevance to the students. (The students were going to be responsible for immunizing people against polio as part of their jobs.)

The test is poor because:

- The students cannot know what information the examiner considers to be important. For example, should they describe the administration of an immunization programme? Should they outline how immunization prevents polio? Or should they describe the side-effects?
- The marking is likely to be unreliable. Because the topic is not clearly defined, different teachers will think different points are more important—and give different marks as a result. Whether a student passes will depend very much on who marks the paper.
- The test is not valid. Students are not going to write essays in their job. They are going to immunize people. Therefore it would be much better to test the skills required for this task.
- The essays will take a long time to mark—if teachers do this job thoroughly.
- The students are unlikely to learn very much from the test.

How could the essay be improved?

The first point is that a different method of assessment would probably be better—some examples are described in the following paragraphs. However, if an essay must be used, you should:

1. Make the title much more specific, for example:

   "Describe how you would explain to mothers why their children should be immunized against polio" or *"Explain how polio vaccine should be transported and given to children"*.

   These essay titles are fairer because it is more clear to students what they should write about. They are also more valid because they ask students to describe the skills that are important.
2. Prepare a marking scheme and follow it. This scheme should include a list of the major points that should be covered in the essay and specify how many marks should be given for accurate

spelling, general clarity of explanation, etc. The scheme should be used by all teachers marking the essay. This improves reliability.

3. After the examination, show the marking scheme to the students and discuss it with them. This helps them to learn.

12.3 Short-answer questions

Short-answer questions allow teachers to ask questions about a larger proportion of the course and to mark more accurately and quickly.

Example of short-answer questions

The following questions were part of an examination for trainee health inspectors.

1. List four advantages to a household of proper rubbish disposal.

(i)
(ii)
(iii)
(iv)

2. Draw a diagram showing the construction of a simple incinerator suitable for use in a small village.
3. Give two examples of situations when burying rubbish is better than composting.

(i)
(ii)

Short-answer questions often ask students to give examples, write down some advantages or draw a diagram. Because they are so much more specific than essays, they are quicker to mark and more reliable. They are also very much quicker to answer. This means that the students can be tested on many more topics during the examination.

The main disadvantage of this method is that it may simply test the students' ability to remember facts rather than apply knowledge or use skills.

12.4 **Multiple-choice questions**

Multiple-choice questions are often called MCQs. They are a stage beyond short-answer questions, because the students do not write any words. They just choose which of several answers is best.

Although you can use four or six choices in multiple-choice questions, five is the most common number. This type of question is sometimes called the *"one-from-five"* type of multiple-choice question.

Example of an MCQ of the one-from-five type

A patient tells you that he is worried because one of his eyes is red. You cannot find any foreign bodies in the eye, but note that the pupil is bigger and does not respond to light. What is the most likely diagnosis?

A. Trachoma
B. Conjunctivitis
C. Iritis
D. Corneal ulcer
E. Glaucoma

In this example, the student has to choose between the possible answers and select the best one—in this case *"E"*. In this type of question, there is a *stem—"A patient tells you . . . likely diagnosis"*—and five choices.

Another type of MCQ is the true/false type.

Example of a true/false MCQ

In glaucoma

A.	There are usually white or grey spots on the cornea.	T. F.
B.	The pupils are irregular.	T. F.
C.	Only one eye may be red.	T. F.
D.	The patient should be referred to a health centre.	T. F.
E.	A foreign body is the most likely cause.	T. F.

Again there is a *stem*—in this example it is very short—"*In glaucoma*".

But this time the stem is followed by several statements. For each statement the student has to decide whether the statement is true or false. In this case "*A*" is false, so the student should draw a circle round "*F*". "*B*" is also false, but "*C*" and "*D*" are true while "*E*" is false, so the student should draw circles round F, F, T, T, and F respectively. In this example the student has to answer all five parts of the question.

Both these types of questions are used fairly commonly, although true/false questions are often preferred because they are easier to understand and can be used to test the students on a wider range of facts.

How useful are MCQs?

MCQs can be marked very quickly and accurately. They can also be answered quickly, so a lot of questions can be set in an examination. This means that a lot of the course can be covered.

On the other hand, there are serious disadvantages. It is quite difficult to write clear questions—so writing the questions takes a lot of time. There is also the very serious problem that MCQs usually only test the students' knowledge. Only rarely do they test decision-making skills and they cannot test the students' ability to communicate or to perform procedures. This means that MCQs are likely to be valid for only a small part of your course.

Despite these problems, MCQs can be useful. They can be used to check factual knowledge, especially during the course. They are also very helpful when used for self-assessment or peer-assessment.

If you decide to use MCQs, the following points may be helpful:

- You should allow roughly 2 minutes for each 5-part true/false question in an examination. So in an hour students can be expected to answer about 30 questions. If you find that students are not finishing the examination, cut down the number of questions. It is not a race.
- For true/false questions, give the students one mark for each correct choice, zero for no answer and take away one mark for each wrong choice.

Use the same scheme for marking one-from-five questions, but do not take away marks for wrong answers.

- The pass mark for MCQs should be quite high. This is because the MCQs should be testing basic knowledge that all students should know. Therefore a pass mark of 80% or 90% can be used successfully. It is better to use easy questions with a high pass mark rather than harder questions with a pass mark of 50% or 60%.
- Marking is made much faster if a separate response sheet is used for the students' answers. Then a mask can be laid over the response sheet, with holes cut out for the correct answers.

Look at the example below. Three correct answers will show through the holes—so you would give 3 marks. There are four ticks

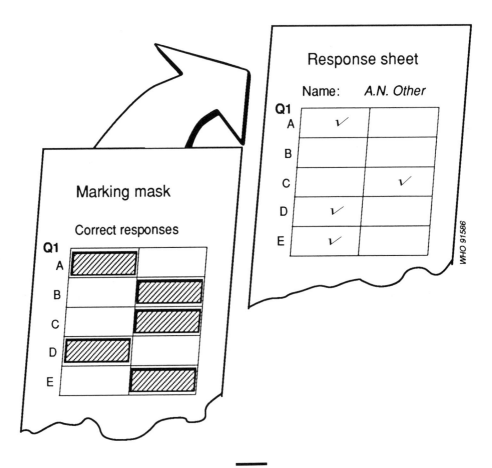

altogether, so one answer must be wrong—so you would take away one mark. This leaves a score of 2 $(3-1)$ for the student.

12.5 Patient-management problems

Patient-management problems are a development of short-answer questions. The main feature is that a series of questions are asked about a case. This method can be used to test students on a wide range of subjects. It can be used wherever students are being trained to make decisions. So it is very useful for assessing students who are training to be health educators, community health workers, community nurses, health inspectors, etc.

Example of a patient-management problem

Mrs A comes to the health centre and tells you that she feels tired all the time. She asks you for a tonic. You find out that she is 30 years old and about 5 months' pregnant.

1. List 3 things that you think might cause the tiredness.
2. Write down 2 other questions that you would like to ask Mrs A.
3. As a result of Mrs A's answers, you suspect she is anaemic. What physical signs would you look for?
4. Your examination confirms your diagnosis of anaemia. What treatment (if any) would you prescribe and what other advice would you give?

This example has the advantages of a short-answer question. It is clear to the student what is required and it will be quick and reliable to mark (providing that all teachers involved agree what the possible causes of tiredness are). It is also much more valid as a test because it is based on the kind of work the students are being trained to do. (It would, of course, be much better if each student met Mrs A and took a history and examined her.) If students are given the marking scheme after the examination, they will also be able to learn from this.

How can you prepare patient-management problems?

It is usually easiest if you base the problem on a case that you have dealt with, such as a boy who presented with severe abdominal pain or a mother who rejected any advice on nutrition, even though her children were malnourished. Of course you can only do this if you still work as a health worker yourself. However, if you teach full-time, talk to health workers or, even better, spend half a day with a health worker to write down examples of cases.

The next stage is to divide the case into stages. What happened first? What decisions had to be made? What alternatives were available?

Then you need to decide what items of information to give the students and what questions to ask them.

At this stage you will have a patient-management problem, but you will still need to develop a marking scheme. List all the answers that you think students might give—both right and wrong. Then decide how many marks you will give for each of the possible answers.

12.6 Project reports

In a number of courses, students are asked to work on a project. This may involve such tasks as doing a survey of a community or working in a health care team for a few weeks. Often the students then present a report on the project and this can take a lot of time.

Naturally students will be more motivated in the project if their reports are assessed and the marks count towards the final examination score.

However, project reports are extremely difficult to mark fairly because there are usually no clear standards for teachers to follow. Some students may do very good work but present a poor report. Others will present a very clear and full report of poor work. Which is best and what standard should you accept?

The following guidelines may help you to assess project work.

1. Project work should be assessed by at least two people marking independently. The two marks should then be compared and discussed to reach a final mark.
2. Where possible, explain to students what standards they should

aim for. Tell the students what you think a good project would be like. Where possible, explain how much data should be collected, how many cases should be seen, and what kind of graphs or tables would be useful. But be careful not to restrict the students too much.

3. Show the students some project work done in previous years that you think is good and also some that you think is bad. Explain your reasons. Of course you cannot do this when you first use projects—so it may be better not to count the marks for the first projects in the overall assessment.

Clearly, the use of projects in assessment causes some problems for the teacher. What is their value? Project reports take a lot of time to mark and the score may not be reliable. However, this method of assessment can be valid if the projects are chosen carefully to involve the students in practising the important skills. Above all, projects can be very powerful learning experiences and they should be assessed to encourage students to make the maximum effort.

12.7 Casebooks

Casebooks have been used quite widely in training nurses and they can also be used in courses for other groups of primary health care staff.

The casebook contains a list of skills or tasks that the students should be able to do. These tasks are the objectives, or at least some of the objectives, for the course. The students are responsible for learning how to do each of the tasks, and when they are ready they can ask a teacher to assess their performance. During the course the students must perform all of the tasks to a satisfactory standard. If the teacher thinks that a student's performance is not good enough, the faults are explained and the student can try again later.

Example—A page from a student's casebook

Task	Date	Signature
17. Prepare a flip chart for use with an audience of 30 people 18. Give advice to a pregnant woman about antenatal care	20/10/90	M. Gunn

This assessment method uses quite a lot of the teacher's time because each student must be seen and his or her performance must be assessed. It can be difficult to organize because teachers may not be available when the student is ready to be assessed. There may be problems with reliability. On the other hand, there are a number of advantages. The main advantage is that casebooks help learning. They do this by making clear to the students what needs to be learned. They also make sure that when students are not up to standard, the teacher is there to give advice. The second advantage is that the method is highly valid, because students are assessed on how well they can do the tasks and jobs that they are being trained to do.

This is a slightly different type of assessment. You do not give students a mark out of ten for each performance—you simply decide whether they are good enough or not. So at the end of the course, a student may have performed 23 out of the 29 set tasks to a satisfactory standard. It is then up to the examiners to decide whether this is a "pass". For some courses, students will need to achieve a satisfactory standard on all the tasks. For others, it may be unnecessary to insist on this high standard.

12.8 Checklists

Checklists are not so much a method of assessment as a way of improving other forms of assessment. Assessments of practical and clinical work are often criticized because the mark is unreliable. Different examiners use different standards. Checklists reduce this problem and they also make sure that the *way* in which the student does the task is assessed.

Example—A checklist for the task "Prepare a thin blood film using a sample of your own blood"

	not done	done correctly
1. Uses middle finger or ring finger		
2. Cleans the finger using surgical spirit or alcohol		
3. Dries finger with a clean piece of cotton wool		
4. Allows blood to flow freely after pricking with needle		
5. Puts a single drop of blood in the middle of the microscope slide		
6. Uses a second slide as a spreader. Allows the blood to spread along the end of the second slide		
7. Pushes spreader quickly along the slide		
8. Draws blood along *behind* the spreader		
9. Does *not* blow on slide or shake it		

The examiner can watch the student preparing the blood film and put a tick in the right-hand column for each part done correctly. At the end of the test, the examiner adds up the number of ticks in the right-hand column and gives the student a score out of 9. The pass mark for this test needs to be decided by the examiner. In this example, the examiner may feel that 7 out of 9 would be a suitable pass standard. For other tests, the examiner might expect 50% or 90%. The pass mark will depend on the specific test.

The advantage of a checklist is that it makes the marking fairer. Different examiners watching a student do a test are more likely to give the same score if they have a checklist. Checklists are also very useful for giving feedback to students or teachers because the evidence is clear and simple. The examiner might tell the teacher *"Most of your students did the blood film test quite well, but I noticed that about half of them pushed the drop of blood instead of drawing it behind the spreader slide"*. This would help the teacher realize that this point needed more emphasis during the next course.

In the same way, detailed information can be given to each student. For example, students might be allowed to see the checklist for their own performance.

The above example is for assessing a psychomotor skill. Similar checklists can be prepared for assessing communication skills and attitudes, but this is often rather more difficult.

Note that you can prepare a checklist from a task analysis.

12.9 In-course assessment

During the training course, your students will probably spend time working in hospitals, health centres or dispensaries. There they will be practising the communication skills and the psychomotor skills needed in their job. This time can be used for assessment as well as teaching.

Many different people will assess the students, so in-course assessment is likely to be more reliable if supervisors are given a checklist to follow. This checklist should be fairly simple, as shown in the example below.

Example—A checklist for assessing students in a health centre

	completely satisfactory	just good enough	not good enough
1. Keeps complete and accurate records			
2. Observes sterile procedures			
3. Establishes good relationships with patients			
and so on			

Nurses or health workers supervising students can use simple checklists to give a clear picture of what the students can or cannot do. You can then use this information:

1. To make decisions on whether students should pass or fail.
2. To give specific advice to students about what they need to learn.
3. To improve the course in areas that are poorly learned.

This kind of checklist is again prepared from a task analysis. Checklists can also be used to help assess attitudes.

Example—A checklist for assessing attitudes

1. Very keen willing worker	├─┼─┼─┼─┼─┤	Does as little work as possible
2. Accepts instructions willingly	├─┼─┼─┼─┼─┤	Resents or ignores instructions
3. Very interested in patients	├─┼─┼─┼─┼─┤	Not interested in patients
4. Always keen to learn	├─┼─┼─┼─┼─┤	Not interested in learning
5. Always on time	├─┼─┼─┼─┼─┤	Always late

This checklist might be used by a senior nursing officer or supervisor on a ward where student nurses spend part of their training. The supervisor would use one form for each student nurse. At the end of the training period, the supervisor would think about the way each of the nurses had worked during their time on the ward.

For example, some nurses might have been quite willing to do what they were asked to do, but never seemed very keen or offered to do extra work. The supervisor would note this down on their forms by putting a cross at about the middle of the line:

1. Very keen willing worker	├─┼─✳─┼─┼─┤	Does as little work as possible

In this way the supervisor can give a fair and quick summary of the attitudes of the student nurses to the teacher responsible for the course. This checklist can be used to give advice to student nurses and can form part of the overall assessment that is used to decide whether they pass or fail the course.

12.10 **Summary**

No assessment method is perfect. Each has some advantages and some disadvantages. You should therefore use a variety of methods whenever possible.

Ideally, you should first decide what skills need to be assessed. These skills are the performance objectives of the course.

Then you should choose the best method for assessing these skills. The method should be chosen on the basis of:

— regulations for the course
— economy of time
— reliability
— validity
— value as a learning tool.

PART
4

Preparing teaching materials

CHAPTER 13

Initial planning

The aim of this part is to help teachers to plan, write, produce, and evaluate materials that will help students to learn. These materials range from single-page handouts which are used in lessons, through to complete manuals which health workers use to help them in their jobs.

This chapter describes the initial planning that must be done. How will the material be used? Who will use it?

Chapter 14 describes ways of writing and evaluating the teaching material.

Chapter 15 explains the use of illustrations and layout.

Chapter 16 gives suggestions about methods of producing and distributing copies of the teaching material.

In each chapter, the first part is aimed at teachers producing material for use in their own classroom or with a small group of students. The second half gives more guidance on methods used in producing manuals for larger numbers of people.

13.1 What are teaching materials?

Teaching materials are any things that help people to learn. In other words, they are materials that teach, such as:

— notes summarizing the main points of a lesson or lecture
— a series of questions which students are asked to answer
— textbooks
— instruction cards for carrying out various tasks
— manuals which help health workers in the field to make a diagnosis.

13.2 Why should teachers prepare teaching materials?

Preparing teaching materials is usually difficult and often takes a lot of time. Why should teachers take on this extra work?
The reasons are:

● Students can learn from the material at any time, so they are less dependent on the teacher.
● Teaching materials help students to learn better.
● Teaching materials can make learning more active (see Section 6.5).

Of course teachers may use teaching materials prepared by other people. For example, many books and manuals have been written specifically for health workers. When these are available and suitable they should be used. But often the books and manuals are written for different categories of health worker or for use in different countries. So teachers often need to adapt these books or even write their own books or manuals for their students.

13.3 Starting to plan the material

Before you start to write any teaching material, there are some questions that you should consider. The questions are given below and then discussed in Sections 13.4–13.8.

Initial planning—A checklist of questions

● Is the material needed?
● How will the material be used?
● Who is the material for?
● Where will the health worker use the material?
● How will you organize the writing and production?

13.4 Is the material needed?

Teaching materials will only be worth writing if they fulfil a need. It is important to decide exactly what the need is, so that the material can be prepared for this specific purpose.

Examples: Situations where teaching materials may help

You may find that you have to explain how to use a particular piece of equipment very frequently. It might be easier to write down the instructions for its use, so that the students can learn how to use the equipment by themselves.

You may find that students find part of the course very difficult. So you could give them some exercises to practise what they have learned during that part.

You might prepare a list of the tasks that you expect students to be able to do. This would guide them and help them to make sure that they had learned all the necessary skills.

You might find that drugs are not being stored properly or they are being prescribed in the wrong doses. Written materials could help to prevent this.

If you find that there is a need for a manual or some other type of written material, you should also check that:

— no other suitable materials are available
— the people who you want to read the material are able and willing to use it.

13.5 **How will the material be used?**

There are different ways in which teaching material may be used. The style of writing, layout, and amount of explanation will all depend on the way in which you expect the health worker to use the material.

1. **Used as training materials.** Materials can be used to present new information or to describe skills that need to be learned by the students. In this case, the material should have detailed explanations, step-by-step instructions, a lot of examples and possibly some exercises.

   Materials like this might be used during the initial training course or to explain new methods of doing a particular task. They might also be used for re-training health workers.
2. **Used as reference materials.** Materials can also be used to

remind health workers about facts or skills that they learned during the training course.

These materials are called reference materials and are often written in the form of a manual.

A reference manual might contain dosages of drugs which the health worker constantly needs to refer to. On the other hand, the manual might contain details of procedures that are only carried out rarely. For example, medical assistants do not have to give advice about the siting of a well very often, so they will probably need to refer to a manual to find out the recommended distances of latrines from a well.

Reference materials must be well indexed so that health workers can find the necessary information quickly. Less explanation is needed because the purpose is to remind them about what they have already learned. Each part of the material must be complete in itself, because the workers will only be using one part at a time — they will not be reading through the book or manual.

Teachers and other people who write manuals should decide what kind of material they want to write at the very beginning. This is because the layout and style are affected by this decision.

13.6 Who is the material for?

Teaching materials must be designed to suit the people who will use them. Therefore you will need to find out about the audience. Below there are some questions that you should be able to answer before you start writing.

How much does the health worker know already?

Ideally, the material should not repeat information that is well known to the health worker. Nor should it assume knowledge that the worker does not have.

This ideal is hard to achieve and quite impossible if health workers come from different backgrounds. If you are in any doubt, it is usually better to assume that they do **not** know something. For example, there is little point in referring to oedema under a list of physical signs if some of the health workers do not understand what the word means. To overcome this problem, talk to some people who will need to use the material so that you can find out exactly how much they know.

How well can the health worker read?

Even though all the people who use the manual will be able to read, they will not be able to read equally well. This is especially important if the language of the manual is not the health worker's mother tongue. So the language and writing style must be simple enough for health workers to understand.

Test the manual with a group of health workers to find out what they understand. For example, this book has been evaluated with groups of teachers to find out whether it can be read easily.

Can the health worker understand the diagrams?

Diagrams are usually used to make an explanation clearer. A good diagram can save hundreds of words and can be remembered more easily. However, understanding diagrams is a skill that is learned, and some health workers may not have developed this skill fully. You should check whether the health workers can understand your diagrams.

Will the health worker have time to read the material?

There is no point in producing long and detailed manuals which are not read. It may be better to write a less complete manual which the health workers have time to use. Alternatively, you could write several shorter manuals instead of one long one. If you do this, the health workers may feel more encouraged to start using at least one of the shorter manuals.

Will the health worker have the time and the resources to do the jobs described?

Sometimes manuals describe jobs that are not realistic. This may be because the health worker has many other jobs to do or because the necessary equipment, medicines or space are not available. If this is the case the manual will not help.

Will the ideas in the material be acceptable to the health worker?

You should take into account the different traditions, and religious and cultural backgrounds of the health workers. For example, a manual describing methods of contraception or sterilization might be of little value if these ideas conflict with their religious beliefs. Workers with other religions or traditions may have objections to other ideas which are good from a purely medical point of view but which conflict with their culture. Ideas such as this require very careful presentation.

13.7 Where will the health worker use the material?

If health workers are taking teaching material (such as a manual) away to their place of work, the explanations must be very detailed because nobody will be available to help them if they are confused. On the other hand, if the manual is to be used where supervision or advice is available, then a briefer explanation may be better.

If students are going to use the material in a training school where they can be helped, then you have much more freedom to use unfamiliar methods of presenting information. For example, you may make more use of diagrams or flow charts.

13.8 How will you organize the writing and production of the material?

When you have decided on the general features of the material, you need to prepare a plan for writing and producing it.

This will not be necessary for handouts or very short material used by one teacher. But when a larger manual or several different people are involved, a plan is essential.

The stages which are often followed are listed below.

Stages in writing manuals and written teaching materials

1. Make the initial planning decisions—as outlined in Section 13.3.
2. Decide on the overall content of the manual and what will be covered in each section.
3. Write out a rough draft.
4. Discuss this with colleagues and some of the people for whom you are writing (e.g. experienced health workers and your students).
5. Rewrite the draft using the layout you want in the final version. Add diagrams, illustrations and index.
6. Evaluate the material.
7. Rewrite the material.
8. Make arrangements for the printing or duplication of the material.
9. Produce and distribute the first edition.

These stages are not rigid. It may be necessary to rewrite the material several times. Additional stages may be required, such as the preparation of training sessions in which the health workers are taught how to use the material. There may be some evaluation at an earlier stage in the process. However, the broad pattern will probably be a useful guide.

A more detailed list of stages is given at the end of Chapter 16.

CHAPTER 14

Writing and evaluating the teaching material

This chapter describes ways of writing and evaluating the teaching material, while Chapter 15 describes how the words should be spaced on the page and how illustrations can be used to make the meaning clearer. Some writers prepare the words and layout at the same time, but for the sake of clarity, these processes are described separately.

14.1 Deciding on the objectives

Manuals and teaching materials are written to help people to do things. For example, one manual called *Obstetric emergencies* is designed to enable rural health workers to treat women with obstetric emergencies and to know when to refer them to hospital. Another much smaller piece of teaching material has the title *Recording the administration of drugs*. In both cases the general purposes of the materials are clear. The purposes were probably decided during the initial planning when the need for the manual or teaching material was identified.

You must then work out exactly what the health worker must be able to do. Which obstetric emergencies should be covered? Exactly how should rural health workers deal with each type of emergency? Probably the best way to do this is to carry out a task analysis of the work. (The author has carried out several task analyses of the work done by teachers of health workers so that this book would be helpful to teachers.)

Task analysis will help you to:

— include all necessary information
— leave out unnecessary information
— give information in the correct order
— describe all situations in decision-making
— avoid vague instructions.

Examples of how task analysis can be used in writing manuals are given in Sections 14.2–14.5.

14.2 Including all necessary information

Teaching materials and manuals should include all the information that the health workers need in order to do a job.

This point may seem obvious, but often manuals do miss out essential steps or facts. Look at the example of poor instructions below and try to find out what information is missing.

Example—Information missing from a manual

Taking a patient's rectal temperature

Follow the four stages described below:

1. Ask the patient to insert the small part of the thermometer into his or her anus. If the patient is a small child or is unable to do this, insert the thermometer yourself.
2. Leave the thermometer in this position for about 2 minutes. If the patient is an adult, he or she should be lying on one side. If the patient is a child, he or she should be lying face downwards and should be held.
3. Take the thermometer out and read up to which mark the line inside the thermometer has reached. If the line is above 37.5 °C the patient is feverish.
4. Clean the part of the thermometer that has been inside the anus with some cotton wool and soapy water. Put the thermometer away in a safe place.

You will probably have noticed that a health worker following these instructions would not:

— lubricate the thermometer
— shake down the mercury in the thermometer.

This error could have been avoided if a task analysis had been done, especially if it had been checked by watching a health worker doing the task.

14.3 **Leaving out unnecessary information**

There is a great temptation for writers to put down everything they know about a subject. This is bad practice because the unnecessary information distracts the reader from the essential facts.

Exercise

Think about health workers who are responsible for storing vaccines. Which of the following facts do they need to know?

1. The definition of an attenuated vaccine.
2. Which vaccines are absorbed on alum.
3. How vaccines are freeze-dried.
4. How long a vaccine will last at room temperature.
5. How long a vaccine lasts in a refrigerator.

You will probably agree that health workers need to know how long each vaccine will last at different temperatures. They do not need to know what *"attenuated"* or *"freeze-dried"* or *"absorbed on alum"* means. Nor is it useful for them to know which of these types of vaccines they are using. Again, task analysis is a good method for deciding whether some information is necessary or not.

14.4 **Giving information in the right order**

When a procedure is being described, the description should follow the order in which the actions are done.

Exercise

Try to rewrite these instructions in a more sensible order.

Instructions for cleaning a wound

Put antiseptic on and around the wound after shaving off any hair round the wound and washing the wound with soap and water.

These instructions would have been written much more clearly as a list.

Instructions for cleaning a wound

1. Shave off any hair round the wound.
2. Wash the wound with soap and water.
3. Put antiseptic on and around the wound.

Often, writing instructions in the wrong order makes them difficult to understand. Sometimes it can be dangerous. Look again at the poor instructions for taking a patient's rectal temperature. What is bad about the order in which the instructions are given?

The patient is asked to insert the thermometer and **then** the instructions say that the patient should be lying on one side (adult) or face-down (child). Obviously the first instruction should be to ask the patient to lie in the correct position. Only then should the thermometer be inserted.

This kind of error is very common and occurs even in respected manuals written by very experienced health workers. It can be avoided by doing a task analysis.

14.5 Describe all situations in decision-making

Sometimes manuals tell health workers what to do in a specific situation, but do not tell them what to do if the situation is a little different.

Example—Some possible situations are not described

1. A patient has been coughing and spitting for a few days

Take the patient's temperature.

1.1 The patient's temperature is less than 38 °C. Other symptoms:

— a runny nose (with a discharge like water or a thicker discharge like milk) *or*
— a sore throat.

Give the patient aspirin for 3 days and tell him or her not to cough on other people (especially children) or spit on the floor.

This manual tells the health worker what to do in two situations when patients have been coughing and spitting for a few days. The two sets of additional symptoms are:

— low fever and a runny nose or
— low fever and a sore throat.

It fails to mention another common situation when, in addition to coughing and spitting, the patient also has:

— low fever with no other symptoms.

A health worker using the manual can therefore come across a common condition that the manual does not cover. The least harmful effect of this will be dissatisfaction with the manual, but more serious effects are also possible, such as failing to recognize possible cases of tuberculosis.

A task analysis of the diagnosis of cough might have shown that all situations were not covered.

14.6 Avoid vague instructions

Vague instructions like *"be careful"* should be avoided. They do not say in what way care should be taken and are therefore a waste of time. Other examples which are commonly used are:

— *"assemble correctly"*
— *"record the weight properly"*.

Example—Vague instruction

Treatment of cough

To treat people with a cough, see *"Respiratory diseases"* on page 25 and tell the people living in your village:

1. To stay at home when they have a cough and runny nose.
2. To take care of the children and old people and to return to the health centre immediately if . . . .

What does it mean to *"take care of the children and old people"*? The health worker may not know what kind of care should be provided and so much more specific advice should be given.

14.7 Structuring the material

This paragraph refers to longer teaching materials such as manuals. The structure of these materials depends on how they are to be used.

For a manual that will be used for reference, the order of the sections is important but it will not be the same as the order in which the pages will be read. This is because the manual will **not** be read like an ordinary book. Health workers will look at the few pages they need and then put the manual away. So it is extremely important to have a good index that helps them to find the part of the manual they need at that particular time.

To make this possible, the manual will probably consist of a series of sections relating to the tasks to be performed, such as:

— treating patients with diarrhoea
— treating patients with respiratory diseases
— treating patients who are pregnant
— developing water supplies
— educating village people about nutrition.

Other ways of organizing sections are:

A. Systems of the body:

— respiratory system
— cardiovascular system.

B. The setting in which the worker will use the manual:

— dispensary
— health centre.

It is important that the structure of the manual is clear to the health workers, and that they can find the information they require quickly.

Manuals used in training will be read through from start to finish, and so the order of the sections is much more important. Points to note are:

1. Early sections should not depend on skills or knowledge covered in later sections.
2. Common techniques such as giving an intravenous injection or bandaging should be described in a separate section. The health worker can then be referred to the relevant section when necessary.

14.8 Writing simply

It is essential that manuals and teaching materials are written so that they can be understood easily. There is no point in writing if health workers find the material so difficult to understand that they are unwilling, or even unable, to read it.

This is particularly important if the material will be translated into another language or if the material is not written in the mother tongue of the health workers. For example, manuals written in English need to be especially easy to understand if the health workers normally talk in a different language. There are also serious difficulties with languages such as English or Arabic because several different levels of language exist. For example, the writer may use a higher form of Arabic than the health worker usually uses.

Some guidelines for writing simply are given below.

Guidelines for writing simply

1. Use of words

(i) Use simple, short, common words **not** complicated, long or unfamiliar ones. For example, use "*tie*" not "*ligate*". Use "*press with your finger*" not "*apply digital pressure*".

(ii) Be careful using idioms. If the manual is for local use then idioms may make it more interesting and "punchy" to read. But health workers from other countries may find it difficult to understand. For example, do you understand what "punchy" means?

(iii) Explain technical words. Where it is essential to use technical words, these should be explained fully and an example given. Then you should make a point of using the word several times so that the health worker can practise using it.

2. *Sentence construction*

(i) Use positive statements. The sentence "*You should avoid negative statements*" means almost the same as "*You should use positive statements*". The use of the negative makes it much more difficult to understand.

(ii) Use active verbs. Health workers will find it easier to understand sentences written using active verbs, for example:

"*Ask the patient whether he or she feels feverish*" is easier to understand than "*the patient should be asked by the health worker whether he or she feels feverish*".

(iii) Do not use pronouns. When pronouns such as "*he*","*she*", "*it*" or "*they*" are used, the health worker has to decide exactly what or who the pronouns refer to. It is often better (but sometimes clumsy) to write out the full noun.

(iv) Use short sentences and paragraphs. Long sentences are difficult to understand. It is often better to rewrite a long sentence as two or more shorter ones. Long paragraphs are also boring and tiring to read. Simply break them down into shorter ones.

You should test what you write to see whether it is sufficiently easy to read. The aim of the testing is to see whether what you write can be understood by the health worker. Methods for doing this are explained in more detail in Section 14.12.

14.9 **Writing**

Everybody finds it very difficult to write. They may have good ideas about what they would like to say, but when they are faced with an empty sheet of paper, they cannot get started.

Different people use different techniques to help themselves. Some examples are given overleaf. None of these techniques is guaranteed to help, but you could try them. If you find that they are helpful, use them.

1. Set a target of so many words or pages for each day.
2. Arrange a meeting for 10 days ahead to discuss what you have written. Then you will have to prepare something for that meeting.
3. Give yourself a reward after doing a certain amount of writing —for example, a cup of coffee or tea.
4. Start anywhere in the manual. Often it is best to start on the part that you find most easy. This at least gets some words down on paper.
5. Do not worry about the quality of what you write. Once you have something written, you can then improve it.

The process of writing is always difficult, but the more you write, the easier it becomes.

14.10 The reasons for evaluation

There are two general reasons for evaluating teaching materials. The first reason is to find out how useful the material is to the health workers. This is called *summative evaluation*. You might use summative evaluation on manuals written by other people to decide whether your students would find them helpful. Or you might use summative evaluation on material you have produced to give other people guidance on how useful the material is.

The second reason for evaluation is to improve the teaching material. This is called *formative evaluation*. You should use formative evaluation on all teaching material you produce (even simple handouts) so that you can improve the quality.

14.11 What should you evaluate?

The basis for evaluation is to find out whether the teaching material achieves its purpose. For example, do students learn better if they use a handout? Do health workers do a better job if they use a manual?

To find out the answers to questions such as these, you should use your experience and look at the teaching materials. Think about the following questions:

- Are the important techniques covered? Are the important points made? Is the content right?
- Is the language used simple enough? Are the diagrams clear?
- Are all instructions correct? Do the methods suggested in the material fit in with current practice for your students?
- Can the health workers understand the instructions? Are they given in the correct order?
- Can the health workers find the information that they need? Is the index suitable?
- Can the health workers do the tasks described when they use the manual or material?

Obviously some of these questions are only appropriate when you are evaluating manuals. But most of the questions apply to teaching materials in general.

14.12 Methods of testing

When you are evaluating teaching materials, you should find out what the health workers think about the materials. You should also observe the students or qualified health workers using the material and find out for yourself whether they can use it. This is called *performance testing*.

For example, a section of a manual or handout describing how to give a patient an injection could be tested by watching a student perform the task. If the student gives the injection correctly, then the manual is satisfactory.

This kind of performance testing can be carried out by asking the health worker to perform specific skills in a test situation. It can also be done by observing health workers working in their normal workplace and seeing whether they follow the method described in the manual.

The manual can also be evaluated by looking at the results over a longer period. Manuals explaining how to convince village people about the need for a good diet can be evaluated by looking at the number of cases of malnutrition and diseases related to poor diet. If the number of cases decreases, then the manual can be considered to be effective. However, if there is no change or the number increases, you need to investigate the reasons and possibly change the manual.

14.13 **When should you evaluate the teaching material?**

Teaching materials and manuals should be evaluated **before** the final version is produced. This will allow you to improve the material before it is widely used.

It may also be useful to evaluate materials after they have been used for some time. If there are important weaknesses a revised version should be produced.

14.14 **Summary**

- Use task analysis:

    — to decide on the objectives of the material.
    — to include all necessary information and leave out unnecessary information.
    — to give the information in the order in which it will be used.
    — to describe all the possible situations.

- Avoid vague instructions.
- Write simply.
- Evaluate all teaching materials—using performance testing whenever possible.

Layout and illustration

The aim of this chapter is to help teachers to design and illustrate their teaching materials. The first part of this chapter is aimed at teachers who are involved in writing booklets or manuals. But the second part, which deals with illustration, applies equally to manuals, handouts and even the chalkboard and overhead projector.

Sections 15.1–15.8 describe the decisions that have to be made in planning a manual or booklet, such as:

— page size
— margins
— headings
— typeface
— use of space.

All these decisions are to do with the layout of the material.

Sections 15.9–15.17 describe different kinds of illustrations that can be used and offer advice on when to use the different methods.

15.1 What is layout?

Layout is the use of spaces, different typefaces, headings, etc. to make the words on a page have more meaning and interest. Page after page full of words with no spaces would be almost impossible to read. So layout is an essential part in the design of any teaching material.

15.2 Page size

The size of page to be used in the handout or manual must be decided first. This controls the amount of space you have available for illustrations and for words. Charts and large tables will need a large page size. Booklets designed for reference in the field should, if possible, be small enough to fit in a pocket. The sizes which are commonly used are called A-sizes. A4 is often used for books and handouts. If you fold a sheet of A4 in half as shown below, you will get two pages of A5 size. If these are folded in half, you will get four pages of A6 size.

There are larger A-sizes (A1, A2 and A3), but these are not suitable for books or pamphlets.

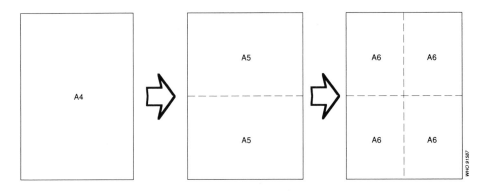

The size of A4 is 297 mm × 210 mm. The ratio of these lengths has been chosen so that when the page is divided into two, the ratio of the long side to the short side stays the same, as shown below:

$$\text{For A4} \qquad \frac{\text{long side}}{\text{short side}} = \frac{297 \text{ mm}}{210 \text{ mm}} = 1.414$$

$$\text{For A5} \qquad \frac{\text{long side}}{\text{short side}} = \frac{210 \text{ mm}}{148.5 \text{ mm}} = 1.414$$

This property allows printers to enlarge or reduce a page produced in the A-sizes to fit exactly any other A-size. For example, if a page of A5 is enlarged by 141%, it will fit A4. If it is reduced by 141% (i.e., to 70% of its original size), it will fit A6.

A5 may be used for reference manuals, and is often used for booklets, since it will usually fit into a pocket. This makes the booklets easy to carry and easy to use for reference—but also means that less information can be included.

Earlier systems of page sizes such as quarto and foolscap are going out of use and should not be used because this will increase the cost of printing the material.

15.3 **Margins**

A margin must be left blank round all the writing and diagrams on the page. This helps to make reading easier because it holds the words in a block. Margins are also useful places for the reader to make notes and increase the usefulness of the book or handout.

The best size of margin is to some extent a matter of taste. For A4 paper the following size is suggested:

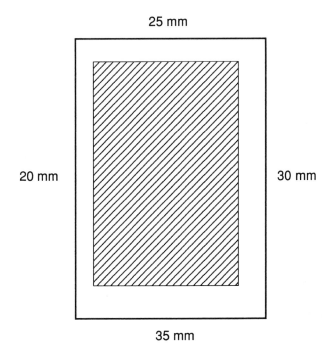

25 mm

20 mm   30 mm

35 mm

WHO 91589

Note: The above example is of a right-hand page. For a left-hand page, the left margin would be 30 mm wide and the right margin would be 20 mm.

However, the modern tendency is to allow larger left-hand margins—as in this book. If you use ring-binding or spiral-binding for a manual, you also need to allow a generous margin along the side that is bound. Otherwise the holes for the binding may pass through text or illustrations.

15.4 **Choice of typeface**

The typeface is the set of letters used in the typewriter or composing machine used by the printer. Most authors will have little choice of typeface because their teaching material will either be handwritten or they will use the only typewriter available. In these cases, the only point to remember is that long strings of CAPITAL LETTERS (which are also called *upper case letters*) are less easy to read than lower case letters. Capital letters should only be used sparingly—for example, in headings.

If the manual is being printed, a much greater choice of typeface will be available. You will need to make choices about:

— size of typeface
— upper case or lower case
— *italic* or roman typeface
— density of typeface (**bold** or normal).

Most of the words will normally be in lower case, roman typeface. The size of typeface is usually 10 pitch or 12 pitch on typewriters. When a composing machine is used, the choice of size is much wider. Common sizes are 10 point or 12 point. The best way to choose the size of typeface is to look at examples of material prepared using different sizes. You should choose a size that is large enough to read comfortably.

If a typeface larger than necessary is chosen, the words will obviously take up more space. In a book, this could mean several extra pages and higher production costs.

If the teaching material is being printed and there is a wide range of typefaces to choose from, you should discuss the use of typeface with the printers and follow their advice.

If you want to emphasize a particular point, you can do this by using upper case letters, a bold typeface or a larger typeface.

However, you should use different typefaces sparingly. You

should **not** use a lot of different typefaces, because this is confusing to the reader. Nor should you use upper case a lot. Upper case is more difficult to read and if all the words are written in upper case none of them is emphasized.

15.5 Use of headings

A solid block of writing on every page is very difficult and boring to read. It is also difficult to use the page for reference. Therefore most teaching materials use headings. These headings:

— break up the text so it is easier to read
— show what the next few paragraphs cover
— help readers to find their place again after they have been looking at a diagram
— help to give the page a pattern.

However, you should only use a few types of heading.

Example—Headings used in this book

This book uses:

— part headings:

PART

4

Preparing teaching materials

— chapter headings:

CHAPTER 15

Layout and illustration

— section headings:

15.1 What is layout?

— subsection headings:

Can the health worker understand the diagrams?

Most books should not need more than about four or five different types of heading. More types only confuse the reader—especially if they are not used consistently.

If you are writing shorter teaching material, then you may only need one or two different types of heading.

15.6 Use of space, lines and boxes

A page of text is divided into paragraphs. This helps to give shape to the page and to make clear to the reader where topics are changed. Space can also be used to emphasize any points that are important. For example, the point made below stands out because of the lines and the space around it.

Use lines and space to emphasize important points.

But do be careful. Too much space is as bad as no empty space. It breaks the continuity of reading and therefore decreases the reader's concentration. Also, if lines or boxes are used all the time they will have less impact. So save lines or boxes for the most important points.

15.7 Use of numbering systems

It is common to number the chapters, sections and even paragraphs of manuals. This has some advantages in making clear to the reader that a new topic is starting and also helps when referring to other sections.

However, the numbering system should be kept fairly simple. In this book, the chapters and sections are numbered. For example, this is Section 15.7. This tells you that it is the seventh section of Chapter 15. Numbering systems which are more complicated than this are not advisable in manuals or teaching materials for health workers.

15.8 Exercise on layout

Exercise

Look at the layout of the double page reproduced overleaf. The layout has some good and some bad features. Make a list of the features that you think are good and those that you would like to improve.

Refer to the previous pages for guidance—then look at the comments below.

Comments

The title "skin diseases" is very clear, because it is large, in a bold typeface and surrounded by a lot of space. This is good. The use of upper case letters might be questioned, but it is satisfactory in a short title such as this.

The section "people who . . . on the skin" is given emphasis by using lines above and below the text. This is good. On the other hand, the use of upper case letters all the way through the two paragraphs means that **all** the words are emphasized equally. They are also more tiring to read. This is poor. There is also no advantage in having the letters in italic script. It would have been better to use lower case, roman letters in a large typeface.

On the second page, the title is given emphasis by the use of upper case letters, underlining and space. This is good.

However, the underlining of "spots", "patches", "blisters", and "scabs" seems unnecessary. The underlining draws attention to these words, but they are not especially important.

LEARNING OBJECTIVES

At the end of his training, the PHW should be able to:

1. find out whether an accident has been the cause of the skin problem

2. decide whether the skin condition covers a small or large area

3. recognize when there is a lump (or a swelling) underneath the skin

4. tell if the skin is covered with red spots, or red patches or blisters or scabs

5. treat a patient who is feverish and has red spots covering a large area of skin

6. treat a patient who is feverish and has blisters and scabs over a large area of skin

7. tell whether a patient has been scratching his skin

8. treat a patient who scratches his skin, when there are no scabs

9. treat a patient who scratches his skin, when a large area of the skin is covered by scabs

10. treat a patient who scratches a small area of his skin

11. treat a patient whose skin is covered with small scabs that have fluid coming out from underneath them

12. decide when a patient with a skin problem should be sent to the hospital or health centre

13. talk with village people about how to prevent skin problems.

S K I N
DISEASES

PEOPLE WHO HAVE SKIN DISEASES BUT NO OTHER SIGNS OF SICKNESS SHOULD WASH THEIR SKIN, COVER IT WITH A MEDICINE AND KEEP THEIR HANDS VERY CLEAN.

PEOPLE WHO HAVE A HIGH TEMPERATURE AS WELL AS A SKIN DISEASE SHOULD BE GIVEN A MEDICINE TO BE TAKEN BY MOUTH OR TO BE INJECTED INTO THE BUTTOCKS AND ANOTHER MEDICINE TO PUT ON THE SKIN.

15.9 **Use of illustrations**

Illustrations such as drawings or pictures can be worth a thousand words of written explanation. They can help to make the explanation clearer and easier to remember. But, if they are not well done, they can also confuse. The following paragraphs describe some of the methods of illustration and give some guidelines on using illustrations effectively.

The various types of illustrations that are described here are:

— photographs
— shaded drawings
— line-drawings
— symbolic or stylized drawings
— cross-sections
— cartoons
— flow charts.

15.10 **Photographs**

Photographs can be very useful for showing students objects and people that cannot be brought into a classroom. They can also be very helpful in books or manuals.

However, photographs are not used very much because of the practical difficulties of obtaining suitable photographs and because they cannot be copied cheaply.

If you want to use photographs, try to choose photographs that have a blank background or else remove the background as shown in the example overleaf. Photo 1 is much clearer than photo 2.

You will also need to use printing—see Chapter 16. This will only be realistic when large numbers of handouts or manuals are required.

15.11 **Shaded drawings**

Shaded drawings may be the most useful way of illustrating a point. The drawing can be prepared to show only those features that are important. Yet they can be realistic enough for the health worker to recognize what is shown.

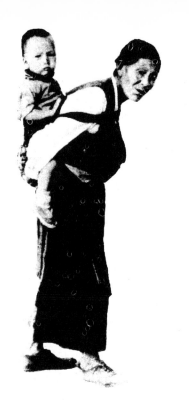

Photo 1

Photo 2

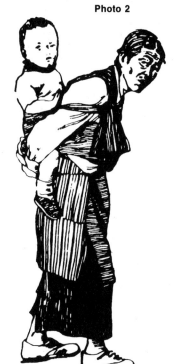

A shaded drawing

162

Shaded drawings can be prepared by tracing a photograph. Another way is to project a photograph onto a white sheet of paper using an epidiascope, then to draw around the projected photograph. This allows enlargement of the original photograph. The results of this process are shown opposite.

Of course, artists can prepare a drawing from real life or from imagination. You can then add labels or notes to it. Look at the example below.

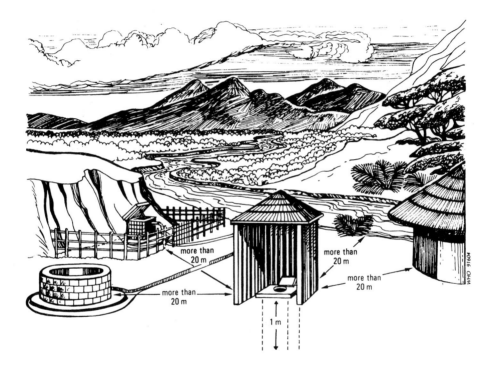

15.12 **Line-drawings**

The figure overleaf is a line-drawing—there is virtually no shading. This kind of drawing is almost as easy to recognize as the shaded drawing and is usually easier to print using a stencil duplicator.

This kind of drawing can be prepared in the same way as shaded drawings.

It looks easier to draw, but often artists say that this kind of drawing requires even more skill than shaded drawings.

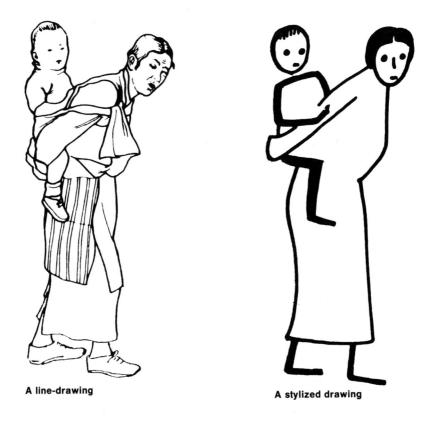

A line-drawing   **A stylized drawing**

15.13 **Symbolic or stylized drawings**

This style of drawing is the easiest to reproduce, but it does require skill in drawing. Also it may not be easily understood by the health workers, so you should always add an explanatory legend or note. For example, look at the stylized drawing above.

15.14 **Cross-sections**

A cross-section is a very useful way of showing what is inside a machine or the human body. But understanding a cross-section is a skill that must be learned. People who are not used to looking at cross-sections will have a lot of difficulty understanding them until they are taught how to do this. For example, the cross-section opposite will be extremely simple for a sanitary engineer who is familiar with cross-sections and the symbols used.

Fig. 36 ANAEROBIC SLUDGE DIGESTION FOR WARM CLIMATES

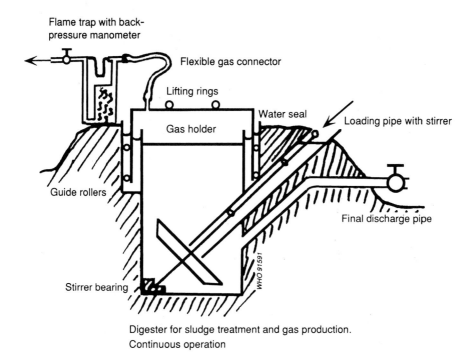

Digester for sludge treatment and gas production.
Continuous operation

On the other hand, a nurse or doctor might find it more difficult to understand, because they might not know what the symbols represent. Students who have not seen cross-sections before would probably also be confused until the diagram was explained to them.

15.15 **Cartoons**

Cartoons are not just funny pictures. The word cartoon is also used to describe line-drawings, especially those showing people saying something.

Cartoons can be very useful for emphasizing important points. They are especially helpful because students are often used to seeing cartoons in newspapers.

The cartoon overleaf helps to make the point more dramatically than a paragraph of words. The words spoken by the people help to make sure that the health workers remember the important points.

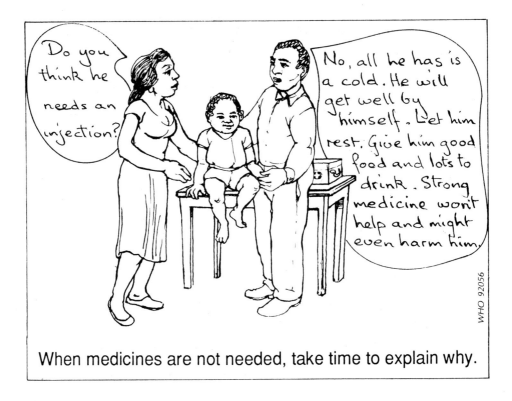

When medicines are not needed, take time to explain why.

15.16 Flow charts

Illustrations are usually thought of as pictures or diagrams. But teaching materials can also be made clearer by using flow charts. These are charts showing what has to be done in different circumstances.

For example, look at the written instructions opposite. You may agree or disagree with the clinical advice given. But the point of the example is that it is rather difficult for the health workers to find out what to do in a specific case. They must go through the whole page to find out how any one patient should be treated.

Example—Written instructions for treating people with a cough

Take the patient's temperature.

1.1 The patient's temperature is less than 38 °C. Other symptoms:

— a runny nose (with a discharge like water or a thicker discharge like milk) *or*
— a sore throat.

Give the patient aspirin for 3 days and tell him or her not to cough on other people (especially children) or spit on the floor.

See the patient again on the 4th day:

— the patient is better. Tell the patient to come back to the clinic if he or she becomes feverish.
— there is no improvement and the patient is feverish—see 1.2.

1.2 The patient's temperature is over 38 °C. Other symptoms:

— difficulty in breathing *or*
— a very sore throat *or*
— discharge from one ear *or*
— red spots all over the body and a runny nose and eyes.

Give the patient penicillin. If penicillin is not available, give the patient sulfadiazine.[a]

See the patient again on the 3rd day:

— the patient is better.
— there is no improvement, send the patient to the hospital or health centre.

---

[a] If you have neither penicillin nor sulfadiazine, send the patient to the hospital or health centre.

Now look at the flow chart overleaf. This gives exactly the same information as the written instructions in a much clearer and more economical way.

Example—A flow chart for "cough"

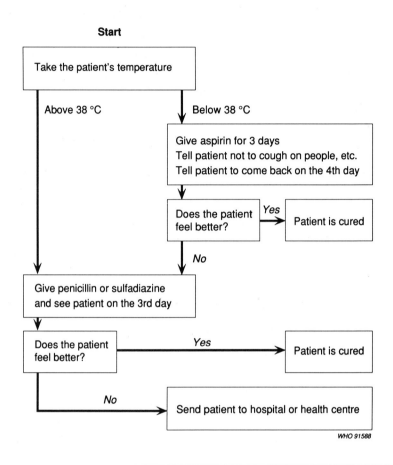

Start

Take the patient's temperature

Above 38 °C   Below 38 °C

Give aspirin for 3 days
Tell patient not to cough on people, etc.
Tell patient to come back on the 4th day

Does the patient feel better?   *Yes* → Patient is cured

No

Give penicillin or sulfadiazine
and see patient on the 3rd day

Does the patient feel better?   *Yes* → Patient is cured

No → Send patient to hospital or health centre

WHO 91588

Flow charts are most useful in handouts or manuals where there is a need to describe a decision-making process, such as deciding what treatment to give patients with certain symptoms.

They are not useful when the task always follows the same sequence: for example, preparing a syringe for injections would not be a good topic for a flow chart.

15.17 **General points**

1. *Students must learn how to read diagrams and pictures*

Pictures are not understood automatically by everybody. People who are not used to looking at pictures just do not understand what they represent. Most students will be familiar with pictures—but the use of diagrams, symbols, cross-sections and flow charts is a skill that must be learned.

2. *Be careful to explain the scale of pictures*

There are a lot of stories about people who are shown pictures of mosquitos and say *"There is nothing like that around here"*. They have not realized that the drawing which is 15 cm long is showing something that is actually less than 1 cm long. This kind of mis-understanding is very common and often occurs when teachers show drawings of objects that can only be seen under a micro-scope.

3. *Test your illustrations*

Find out whether your students really do understand the illustra-tions. Several studies have shown that health workers often do not realize what an illustration is meant to show.

For example, most health workers will understand that the message of this illustration is that drugs and tablets can be danger-ous. They will remember the message well because it is drawn in a dramatic way, using the gun as a symbol of danger, and compares tablets with bullets.

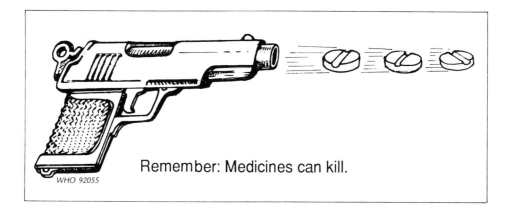

Remember: Medicines can kill.

WHO 92055

However, some health workers might just see a gun and some tablets. Others may not even recognize the gun.

So you must test what the health workers understand and remember from the illustrations.

4. *Keep illustrations simple*

Only show the things that are necessary. Too much detail can distract readers and confuse the point of the illustration.

Simple illustrations will be easier to reproduce.

For example, this illustration shows the important points, but it is still very simple to draw and copy.

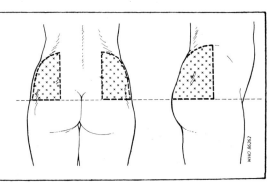

Where to give an injection

It is preferable to inject in the muscle of the buttocks, always in the upper outer quarter.

15.18 **Summary**

1. Layout is very important. It helps the reader to understand the words and helps to emphasize the most important points. Think about:

   — page size
   — margins
   — use of space
   — headings
   — typescript.

   All these things must be used to help the reader learn from the teaching material.

2. Illustrations make teaching material and manuals more effective—if they are used correctly.
3. Check that readers can understand the illustrations that you use.

CHAPTER 16

Production and distribution of teaching materials and manuals

Teaching materials can be produced using very simple equipment and at very little cost. On the other hand, some manuals are very expensive to produce and require sophisticated printing machinery. The choice is yours. Some methods of producing teaching materials and manuals are described below.

16.1 Dictation

Teaching materials **can** be dictated by the teacher. The students simply write down what the teacher says. The disadvantages are that this method requires a lot of time and it rules out the use of diagrams. But the method is the cheapest possible in terms of the materials needed and can be used anywhere. However, dictation is **not** recommended because it takes up too much time.

16.2 Copying from the board

This is much the same as dictation, but allows the use of diagrams. The only resource needed is a chalkboard.

A further advantage is that the layout can be controlled to some extent, but remember that the chalkboard may not be the same shape as the page. Again, this method is **not** recommended because it takes up too much time.

16.3 Stencil duplicator

In this process you write on a master sheet or stencil using a special metal-tipped pen. This pen, called a stylus, removes wax from the stencil. Then you place the stencil on an inked roller and the ink is forced through the gaps in the wax onto the page.

A typewriter can be used to write on the stencil. This is generally more successful than using a stylus. However, if you wish to include diagrams, you will need to use a stylus.

It is difficult to draw pictures or diagrams, but quite possible. A *stencil cutter* may be available. This will allow you to prepare a high-quality stencil from a line-drawing prepared on ordinary paper.

Advantages

— The costs of paper and ink are fairly low (there is no need for high quality or chemically treated paper).
— Many copies (at least 500) can be produced with no loss of quality.
— The stencils can be stored for use the following year (some teachers do this quite successfully; others find that the stencils are difficult to keep in good condition).
— The quality of print is usually good.
— Electrically powered or hand-operated duplicators are available.

Disadvantages

— Only one colour (usually black) can be printed at a time.
— The stencil duplicator is fairly expensive to buy—but much cheaper than printing machinery or photocopiers.
— Some people find stencil duplicators difficult to use.

16.4 Photocopying

The main advantage of photocopying is its convenience. Almost any original can be placed on the machine and a good quality copy produced in seconds. However, the machine is expensive to buy or rent and there are usually extra charges made for each copy. In comparison with offset printing (Section 16.6), the first few copies are usually cheaper, but a large number of copies usually cost much more.

Advantages

— Generally good reproduction of printing or diagrams.
— No limit to the number of copies.
— The originals are easy to prepare.
— Easy to use.
— The copies are available immediately.

Disadvantages

— More expensive than other methods—except for a very small number of copies.
— Poor reproduction of photographs.
— Certain colours cannot be reproduced—for example, light blue.
— Equipment requires good standard of maintenance.

16.5 **Word processing and desk-top publishing**

Over the past few years, computers have become very much cheaper, more reliable and easier to use. It is now possible to buy a sophisticated personal computer for not much more than a good quality typewriter.

In many countries, this means that it is now possible for training schools to purchase a personal computer. Computers can be used by training schools in a number of ways, as discussed below.

The most common use is as a word processor. When used in this way, the computer acts like a very sophisticated typewriter that can remember hundreds of pages of text. This leads to several advantages:

● If a mistake is found or a change is needed, only the change needs to be typed in. Everything that is unchanged is remembered by the computer and retyped automatically. This encourages teachers to improve handouts and teaching materials each year.
● Because it is easy to correct mistakes, teachers find it easier to type their own teaching material. They are less dependent on secretaries.
● Word processors have many other features. For example, they can be used to check the spelling of most words. They also give you

173

much more control over typeface and layout, so documents look better and are easier to read.

The document is stored as a file in the computer. When all the corrections have been made and the layout is satisfactory, the document can be printed using a dot matrix printer (fairly cheap and reasonable quality of printing) or a laser printer (more expensive and better quality of printing).

Desk-top publishing is the name given to a more sophisticated kind of word processing. To use desk-top publishing, you need a reasonably sophisticated personal computer, a laser printer and the appropriate software. The advantages of desk-top publishing over ordinary word processing are that more sophisticated graphics can be used and there is more flexibility over the use of typefaces and layout. However, this also means that you need to have a good knowledge of layout and illustration.

At present, few training schools have the equipment for these techniques. However, the advantages of these methods, combined with steadily decreasing costs and high reliability, mean that more and more training schools will use the techniques in the future.

16.6 Offset printing

There are two main kinds of printing—*offset* and *letterpress*. Offset printing (also called lithographic or litho-printing) has many advantages over letterpress.

In offset printing, the original page or drawing is photographed to make a "printing plate". This plate is then put into the printing machine. The machine prints onto plain paper, giving a high quality at a fairly low cost. When many copies are needed or when photographs are required, this is the best method of producing teaching materials or manuals.

Advantages

— High quality of reproduction.
— Very large number of copies possible.
— Cheap, especially for long print runs.
— Photographs and shaded drawings can be printed.

Disadvantages

— The equipment is expensive.
— A trained technician is required to operate and maintain the equipment.

Summary—Choosing the method of production

The best method of production depends on the number of copies, the quality you require, and the equipment available.

If you are preparing a one- or two-page handout for a few students, use the stencil duplicator. Photocopying might be useful if you want to copy diagrams from a book (with the author's and publisher's permission), but this method is expensive and is rarely available. If you cannot use any of these types of equipment, write your own notes and make carbon copies for the students to copy in their own time.

For longer documents or a larger number of copies, you need to use the stencil duplicator or offset printing. Offset printing is generally better, but if it is not available, the stencil duplicator gives satisfactory results.

16.7 Proofreading

Proofreading is the process of checking the original or "proof" before it is printed. All teaching materials or manuals must be carefully proofread before they are distributed. An error in a manual could lead to injury or loss of life—so the greatest care **must** be taken.

Proofreading is necessary before copying the original manuscript and at a second stage if the material is printed. If the material is printed, it should be checked in the draft form before it is sent to the printers. The printer will then send proofs to you to be checked. It is essential that at both these times **all** errors are found. If errors are discovered later, it may be impossible to correct them and will certainly be expensive.

The worst people for proofreading the material are the people who have written it. They tend to miss errors because they know what should be there. So choose at least two other people who are thorough and careful to read the final draft or proof for you.

You must allow enough time for proofreading. If it is done in a hurry, there is much more chance of missing errors.

16.8 **Distribution**

If the teaching material will be used by your own students, then you can simply hand it out in the classroom. But if the material is a manual for health workers in the field, you must plan how to distribute it.

When the teaching material or manual has been printed, it must be distributed to the people you want to read it. You should not simply put the manual in the post and hope that it will be read by the health workers. If you do this, then health workers will often not even open the material or may just glance at it before putting it away on a shelf.

The best method of distribution will depend on local circumstances and the amount of time and resources available. However, you can encourage health workers to read the manual by using some of the following ideas:

- Write a letter to the health workers, explaining why the manual will be useful to them. It will help if the letter is addressed to the health workers by name and signed by their teacher or supervisor.
- Invite comments on the manual to show that you are interested in the health workers' opinions.
- Arrange a meeting where a group of health workers can discuss the manual. This may be done as an introduction to the manual or it may take place about a month after the manual is sent out.
- Arrange for supervisors to deliver the manual personally. They can then explain to the workers why the manual is useful.
- Arrange workshops in which the manual or teaching materials are used. Then allow the workers to keep the manual at the end of the workshop.
- Do anything that will encourage the health workers to open the manual and start to use it.

16.9 **Summary of Part 4**

A checklist is given below, summarizing the whole of Part 4. It is based on a checklist used in India by a group who produce manuals for health workers. It is aimed at people who write manuals rather than teachers who produce a few handouts. But the checklist will still be useful (even though some of the questions are unnecessary) for anyone producing any teaching material.

You should not follow this checklist rigidly. Instead, read through it and use it as a guide. Sometimes you may want to follow the stages in a slightly different order. Or you may leave out some of the stages. However, the checklist should provide a useful reminder of the stages.

Checklist for preparing and distributing manuals

1. Decide on the category of health workers for whom the manual is to be prepared.
2. Decide on the language in which the manual is to be written and whether it is to be translated into other languages.
3. Decide who is to prepare the manual:

   — one person?
   — a team of two or three people, with one person acting as coordinator and general editor?
   — several contributors? In this case, one person should act as coordinator and general editor to ensure conformity of style and to assign the topics that need to be covered. Each contributor should be given a list of instructions regarding content, length of chapters, general format, etc.

4. Familiarize yourself with the health organization in which the health workers will work.
5. List the tasks that the health workers will need to be able to perform.
6. Analyse the tasks.
7. List:

   — the information required to be able to do the tasks
   — the skills required for carrying out the tasks
   — the stages involved in the tasks (the sub-tasks)
   — the points for health education.

8. Decide on the format of the manual

   (i) Parts, chapters, sections, subsections, annexes.
   (ii) Whether the manual is to be written as a series of chapters on:
       — tasks
       — topics
       — systems of the body.
   (iii) Title of the manual.

    (iv) Style of writing:
- formal
- informal
- use of "you" or "the worker".

    (v) Inclusion of:
- cross-sectional diagrams
- photographs
- line-drawings
- shaded drawings
- symbolic or stylized drawings
- cartoons (black and white/colour)
- flow charts
- tables.

9. Collect existing literature and documents used for education and training in the various health programmes and discuss the topics with the programme officers concerned.

10. Write or type the draft chapters:

- outline each chapter, then fill in details
- write in sequence starting with chapter 1, or start with whichever chapter is easiest.

11. Decide what illustrations need to be included in each chapter. Collect references for illustrations. Prepare diagrams, photographs, cartoons, etc. List the captions.

12. Discuss relevant chapters with programme officers and check for accuracy of facts, figures, illustrations, etc.

13. Prepare a chapter of instructions for the health workers on how to use the manual.

14. Prepare the list of contents and index.

15. Prepare the foreword and acknowledgements.

16. Read through the whole manual to check for continuity and completeness. Edit and rewrite where necessary.

17. Decide on the style for typing and give instructions to typist regarding spacing, boxes, flow charts, headings, numbering of chapters, insertion of illustrations, etc.

18. Prepare final typescript according to instructions.

19. Check typescript against original manuscript.

20. Decide on style of manual and copy-edit typescript accordingly. Pay attention to punctuation, abbreviations, numbering, typeface used for text, chapter headings, headings and

subheadings, and instructions for insertion of illustrations, tables and flow charts.

21. Discuss the layout and design of the manual with a graphic designer:

— cover design and colour
— binding
— size of manual
— page format (full page or columns)
— right-side justification
— printing process (e.g. offset or letterpress)
— typeface, etc.

Clear instructions in writing regarding the style decided upon should be given to the designer as well as to the printer.

22. Decide on the number of copies to be printed, based on intended distribution. Work out costing. Obtain financial approval or aid from other sources.

23. Call for tenders. Select a printer on the basis of:

— finances available
— quality of work
— process and type of printing available
— time constraints
— convenience.

24. Send edited typescript to printer. When proofs arrive, check immediately.

Galley proofs

— compare with typescript
— read through
— mark any corrections needed
— check continuity of numbering of pages, paragraphs, etc.

Page proofs

— check that all corrections in galley proofs are made
— read through
— mark any further corrections needed.

Paste-ups/blueprints (offset) or final page proofs (letterpress)

— check that all corrections in page proofs are made

— read through
— check continuity of numbering
— make sure that text and illustrations, etc. are not broken at inappropriate points
— check page headings, including page numbers and section numbers used
— check that illustrations, flow charts and tables are in the right places and check figure numbers and captions (If offset printing or printing blocks are used, be careful to see that illustrations are not reversed or placed upside down.)
— mark corrections on paste-ups in soft pencil in the margins. Do not disfigure or dirty the paste-ups.

25. Prepare a distribution list of names and addresses of institutions and individuals, together with the number of copies to be sent to each. Check that a sufficient number of manuals is kept in stock.
26. Arrange for the receipt of printed copies and for storage and preservation from insects and rodents.
27. Arrange for packing and dispatch of the manual.
28. Decide on method of evaluating the manual.
29. Carry out evaluation of the manual, based on postal questionnaires, interviews, observations, tests, etc.
30. Invite comments and suggestions from health workers on ways of improving the manual.
31. Revise the manual, basing your revision on:

— results of evaluation
— comments and suggestions received
— up-to-date information to be supplied to workers
— changes in policy.

Note

The steps listed may not be followed exactly in the sequence in which they have been arranged. This list can serve as a checklist of things to be done in preparing a manual. It is based on the experiences of people involved in preparing manuals for health workers and community health workers under the Rural Health Scheme of the Indian Government.

This checklist is reproduced with the permission of the Training Division of the Ministry of Health and Family Welfare, Government of India.

Explanation of terms used in this book

academic discipline   A branch of instruction or learning, such as anatomy, physiology, ophthalmology or history.

active learning   The way in which students learn by doing things, such as solving problems, doing a project or working in a health centre. Sitting listening to a lecture or reading a book is not active learning (Section 6.5).

assessment   The process of testing a student's ability or skill. This may be done in an examination or by more informal methods.

attitude   A tendency to behave or think in a certain way. For example, one health worker may refuse to see patients when the health centre is closed. Another may be willing to see patients at any time. This is because they have different attitudes to their job.

book learning   The kind of learning that can be achieved by reading books. The phrase is usually used to imply that what is learned is too theoretical and not sufficiently practical to be useful.

case history   The information about a patient that is used in treatment. It includes details of the patient's symptoms, the results of any tests or examinations performed, and treatment.

cognitive   Associated with thinking (see also skill).

communication   The process of transferring information or skills to other people. For communication to take place, a *message* must be sent by one person and received by the other. Communication is not just a matter of speaking or writing. It also involves listening to and accepting other people's opinions and beliefs. Skills in communication are very important in health care (see skill).

community   A group of people who live in the same geographical area such as a village or part of a city. The word can also be used to refer to a group of people who have something in common, such as a religion or a profession.

critical incident studies   Studies of events or situations that trained health workers have not felt able to handle. By analysing these incidents, the teacher can find out where more training is required.

curriculum   The written description of what happens during a course. It describes the objectives of the course, the teaching methods, the amount of time allotted to each part of the course, and the methods to be used to assess the students. The word curriculum is also used to describe what actually happens during the course (which may not be the same as the written curriculum).

curriculum design   The process of planning a curriculum for a course. Briefly, this involves deciding:

— what the students need to learn;
— what teaching methods will be used;
— how students will be assessed;
— the time and place where students will learn (the timetable).

evaluation   The process of collecting information about assessing the value of a course, a book, a lesson or even a student. Evaluation may be used to improve the quality of the course or teaching material. This type of evaluation is called formative evaluation. Evaluation may also be used to describe and assess the overall value of the course or teaching material. This is called summative evaluation.

facilitator   A person who makes things easier. For example, a teacher should be a facilitator of learning—i.e., the teacher should make it easier for students to learn.

feedback   The process of telling people how well they are doing. For example, teachers give feedback to students whenever they comment on the quality of the students' work. Ideally, the teacher should point out how well the work has been done, any errors or faults, and how the quality could be improved (Section 6.6).

field experience   Experience of doing the job in the community. Trainee health workers often join qualified health workers for periods of attachment. In this way they gain experience of doing the job for which they are being trained. The students work under supervision, and are given feedback on their performance (see feedback).

health care team   A group of people who provide health care in a community. This may include a midwife, a nurse, a health inspector, a health educator, a nutritionist, a health extension officer, and/or a doctor.

job description   A description of the work that a particular category of health worker is expected to do. It usually consists of a list of the tasks to be done, such as "*measure blood pressure*" or "*select sites for wells*". It may also describe the conditions under which the work will be done.

learning   The process of acquiring information or skills. For example, students can learn from reading books or manuals, listening to lectures, and practising what they have been taught (see active learning).

learning experience   Anything which happens to a student that helps him or her to learn. For example, a student might visit a village where the people have improved the water supply. If the student learned how other villages could do the same, this would be a learning experience.

lesson plan   The set of notes that teachers write to guide themselves as they give a lesson. The lesson plan might include the main points to be covered in the lesson, activities for the students to do, questions related to the topic being taught and some form of assessment.

manual   A book that describes in detail how to do various tasks. The word manual is now often used to describe any book that provides information.

MCH clinic   A maternal and child health clinic. The staff are responsible for checking the growth and health of children and mothers and for providing preventive health care (see preventive health care).

mother tongue   The language spoken by a person at the time when he or she first learns to speak.

motivation   Interest or drive which causes a person to behave in a certain way. For example, a student with a strong motivation will tend to work hard and learn quickly. Motivation is also used to describe the process of encouraging or "motivating" a person. For example, motivation occurs when a student is inspired or persuaded to study hard. This may be because the teacher has made the course more interesting, easier to learn, or more relevant to the job (Chapter 6).

objective   The target or goal of teaching. For example, when the students have completed the course, they should be able to do tasks such as "*construct a latrine*" or "*teach mothers how to breast-feed a baby*".

patient-management problem   An exercise based on a case report, which can be used to help students to learn (as a basis for discussion or in self-assessment) or as a method of assessment. Briefly, the students are given some information about a case and are then asked to answer a series of questions (see Section 12.5).

peer   A person who is of the same ability or standing. For example, a student's peers are the other students on the course. A teacher's peers are the other teachers.

preventive health care   Health care designed to prevent people becoming ill, rather than to cure them once they are ill. Examples of preventive health care include immunization, education, monitoring growth of children, and eliminating sources of disease.

reference materials   Books, records, notes, tables or other sources of information used by students or health workers in order to find factual information.

reliability   A measure of the accuracy and consistency of the marking of tests or examinations. For example, if a student was given a mark of 75% by one examiner and 50% by another examiner for the same performance, the reliability of the marking would be poor.

resources   Anything that is needed to do a job. For example, some of the resources needed for running a course are a classroom, teachers, and writing materials.

self-assessment   The process of testing and judging one's own performance. For example, a student who attempts some problems, then looks up the answers to see how well he or she has done is using self-assessment. Self-assessment can help students to learn.

situation analysis   The process of finding out exactly what a health worker should do in his or her work. This leads to a list of all the tasks done by the health worker.

skill   The ability to perform a task through the application of knowledge and experience. There are different kinds of skills. For example, cognitive skills are skills of thinking such as making decisions or reaching a diagnosis. Psychomotor skills are skills of coordinating the mind and body. For example, stitching a wound is a psychomotor skill—deciding whether stitching is appropriate is a cognitive skill. Communication skills are the skills of talking, explaining, persuading and listening.

syllabus   A written description of what should be learned by the students in a course. Usually it is a brief statement outlining the topics to be covered.

task   Anything that a person does as part of his or her job. For example, a health inspector may investigate water tanks to find out whether they could be breeding sites for mosquitos.

task analysis   The process of studying a task in order to find out exactly how the task is done and exactly what knowledge and attitudes are needed in order to do the task.

teaching materials   Materials that help students to learn, such as books, handouts, models, exercises, and written questions.

trainee   A person who is being trained. For example, a trainee health worker is a person who is being trained to be a health worker.

typeface   The style of lettering. If teaching materials are printed, there is usually a wide choice of typefaces available. The typeface can vary in size, boldness and style. For example, the letter "a" may be printed as an italic "*a*" or in various styles of roman lettering e.g. "a".

validity   A measure of the usefulness of tests or examinations. A test is valid if it really does test the kinds of skill or knowledge that the students need in order to do a job. For example, if a teacher wants to find out whether students can measure blood pressure, he or she might ask them to write an essay on "*The reasons for measuring blood pressure*". This would not be valid. A valid test would be to ask the students to measure a patient's blood pressure and to watch them doing the task.

visual aid   Anything that is used to show a diagram or picture. For example, if a teacher wants to explain an idea to the students, he or she will often draw a diagram or picture on the blackboard or chalkboard, or show photographs, films, or flip charts, etc.

workshop   A meeting at which a group of people learn together. Often they will meet to discuss and solve a specific problem. Sometimes the workshop is more like a short course in which the participants discuss problems, attempt projects, and learn skills.

Index